SMILE A MILE MORE
THE LIBRARY OF ALL THE QUERIES OF THE DENTISTRY

DR SWATI CHAUDHARY

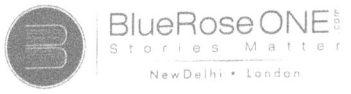

BLUEROSE PUBLISHERS
India | U.K.

Copyright © Dr Swati Chaudhary BDS MBA HA 2023

All rights reserved by author. No part of this publication may be reproduced, stored in a retrieval system or transmitted in any form or by any means, electronic, mechanical, photocopying, recording or otherwise, without the prior permission of the author. Although every precaution has been taken to verify the accuracy of the information contained herein, the publisher assumes no responsibility for any errors or omissions. No liability is assumed for damages that may result from the use of information contained within.

BlueRose Publishers takes no responsibility for any damages, losses, or liabilities that may arise from the use or misuse of the information, products, or services provided in this publication.

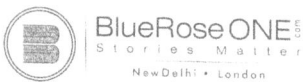

For permissions requests or inquiries regarding this publication, please contact:

BLUEROSE PUBLISHERS
www.BlueRoseONE.com
info@bluerosepublishers.com
+91 8882 898 898
+4407342408967

ISBN: 978-93-5819-387-9

Cover design: Shivam
Typesetting: Namrata Saini

First Edition: August 2023

Acknowledgement

This book compiles an introduction to the basic knowledge of dentistry, and various specialties in dentistry. It is aimed at educating the masses about various diseases/conditions that may affect the oral cavity and provides a guide on how to approach the dental fraternity for the required treatment.

This book will help create awareness among the general masses regarding the importance of oral health and guide them in achieving it. It will aid them in understanding which specialist to seek for their treatment needs.

The book will be able to bridge the gap between the dentist and the patient, as the patient will be able to understand better the treatment rendered to them.

Preface

It has combined information on all dental specialties under one umbrella. It acts as a comprehensive guide for the common masses based on all general queries that they may have and general awareness issues regarding oral health and diseases.

This compilation has the potential to be beneficial to the public as well as professionals.

This book can serve as a tool in giving the basic idea of all the specialties and the unique options rendered.

The knowledge and information provided here will help the patients to safeguard themselves from quacks and unethical practices.

Acknowledgement

This book compiles an introduction to the basic knowledge of dentistry, and various specialties in dentistry. It is aimed at educating the masses about various diseases/conditions that may affect the oral cavity and provides a guide on how to approach the dental fraternity for the required treatment.

This book will help create awareness among the general masses regarding the importance of oral health and guide them in achieving it. It will aid them in understanding which specialist to seek for their treatment needs.

The book will be able to bridge the gap between the dentist and the patient, as the patient will be able to understand better the treatment rendered to them.

Preface

It has combined information on all dental specialties under one umbrella. It acts as a comprehensive guide for the common masses based on all general queries that they may have and general awareness issues regarding oral health and diseases.

This compilation has the potential to be beneficial to the public as well as professionals.

This book can serve as a tool in giving the basic idea of all the specialties and the unique options rendered.

The knowledge and information provided here will help the patients to safeguard themselves from quacks and unethical practices.

Foreword

SMILE A MILE MORE is a comprehensive mini manual book that deals with all the queries of dentistry. However, it has been detailing the ways and means of collecting scientific information and its application in the diagnosis and management of oral health. This mini-book fulfils the need to a large extent. The manual is specifically prepared to aware the general public of the society.

However, emphasis is laid on the oral health of the general public. The manual will be very useful and handy for day-to-day reference.

Contents

Introduction 1

History of Dentistry 2

Branches of Dentistry... 5

Principles of Ethics.. 6

Dental council of India 7

Origin.. 8

Important Days 9

Anatomy of Tooth 10

Different Parts of a Tooth... 11

Different Types of Teeth? 12

Dentition 13

Functions of the Tooth and the Oral Cavity 16

Tips for Better Dental Health... 17

Dos and Don'ts 18

What problems could Poor Dental Health Cause? 19

Do You Feel Nervous about the Dentist?...................... 20

Tips for Easing Dental Fears 22

Overcoming Fear with Prevention.................................. 23

Habits That Ruin Your Teeth 24

How Often Should You Visit the Dentist? 28

Who Should Go to the Dentist More Often?................. 29

Why is Going to the Dentist Important? 30

What Can You Do to Keep Dentist Appointments to a Minimum? 31

Oral Health for Diabetics 32

Oral Medicine & Radiology 36

    Supportive Investigations 37

    Why Dental X-Rays Are Performed 38

    Common Dental Radiography 38

        Intraoral X-Ray 38

        Extraoral X-Ray 40

    Few Common Lesions 42

    Oral candidiasis (Thrush). 42

    Leukoplakia- What is leukoplakia? 46

    OSMF Oral submucous fibrosis. 48

    Oral Cancer 52

Periodontology 59

    Gingivitis 60

    Dental Plaque 63

    Tartar (Dental Calculus) 65

    Tooth Discoloration- 69

Orthodontics 76

    Benefits of Orthodontics 76

    Removable Appliances 78

    Fixed Appliances 79

Oral and Maxillofacial Surgery 82

    Tooth Extraction 83

    10 Things You Did Not Know About Wisdom Teeth! 86

Pedodontics 89

- Natal/ Neonatal Tooth 93
- Nursing Bottle Caries/ Early Childhood Caries 94
- Ugly Duckling Stage 94
- Cleft Lip and Cleft Palate 95

Conservative and Endodontic Dentistry 99
- Dental Caries/ Tooth Decay/ Cavity 102
- Restoration / Fillings 103
- Amalgam Restorations 103
- Composite Restoration 104
- Glass Ionomer Cement Restoration 105
- Gold Restoration 106
- Root Canal Therapy (Rct) 107
- Dental Bleaching 109

Prosthodontics 111
- Missing Tooth and Its Effects 112
- Causes of Tooth Loss / Tooth Replacement Options .. 113
- Dental Crown / Cap 115

Oral Pathology 118

Public Health Dentistry 120
- What Is In Toothpaste? 120
- Which Toothbrush To Use / Toothbrush Selection 123
- Toothbrushing 125

Lasers in Dentistry 128

Handy Tips 129
- Sore Throat 130
- Sensitive Teeth 130
- Dry Mouth 131
- Avulsed Tooth 131

Salt Water Rinse	133
Pregnancy and Dental	**134**
Mouthguards: Things You Need To Know	**135**
Interesting Teeth and Dental Facts That Will Surprise You	**137**

Introduction

DENTISTRY-Dentistry is defined as the evaluation, diagnosis, prevention, and/or treatment (non-surgical, surgical, or related procedures) of diseases, disorders, and/or conditions of the oral cavity, maxillofacial area and/or the adjacent and associated structures and their impact on the scope of his/her education, training and experience, in accordance with the ethics of the profession and applicable law (as adopted by the 1997 American dental association house of delegates). It comprises various specialties and sub-specialties and the specialist of each field is known for their specialization.

DENTIST- One whose profession is to treat diseases and injuries of the teeth and oral cavity and to construct and insert restorations of and for the teeth, jaws, and mouth.

History of Dentistry

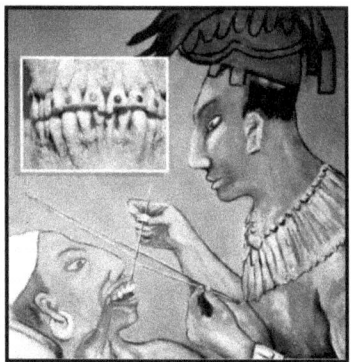

Silver amalgam restorations in the ancient times

- Roots of dentistry can be traced back to ancient times, as early as 200 BC in China, India, and, Japan where silver amalgam was used as filling material.
- Tooth extraction was practiced in Greece at the time of Hippocrates around 400 BC
- Dental bridges and partial dentures of gold have been found in Etruscan tombs that date to about 500 BC.
- Accounts of dental treatment have appeared in Egyptian scrolls dated as far back as 1500 BC

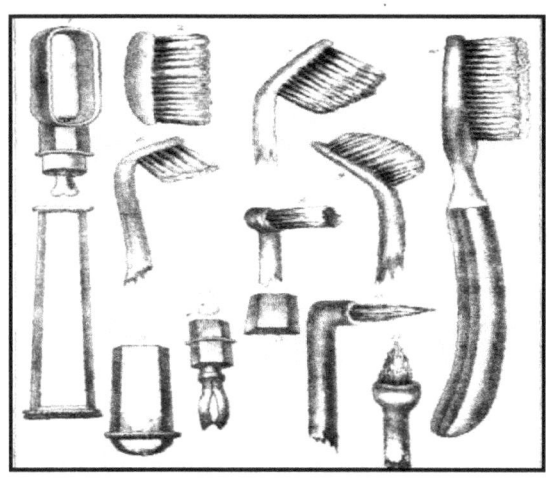

Oral cleaning aids used in the ancient times

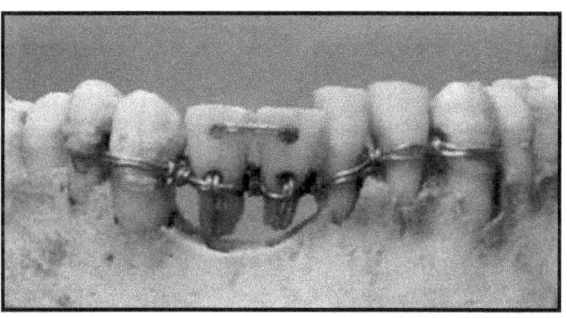

Tooth reimplantation used before introduction of prosthetic materials

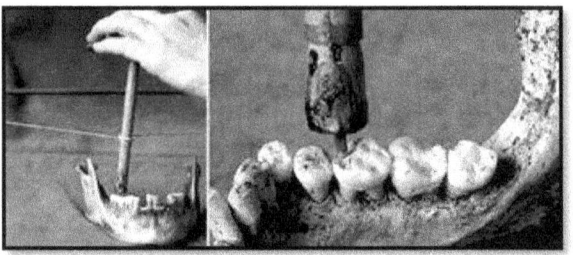

Cavity preparation in the ancient times

Abbreviations-

Dr - Doctor

B.D.S – Bachelor of Dental surgery.

M.D.S. – Master of Dental Surgery.

Tooth Enamel Is The Hardest Part Of The Body.

Branches of Dentistry

- ✓ Oral Medicine and Radiology
  (Oral Radiologist)
- ✓ Orthodontic and Dentofacial Orthopedics
  (Orthodontist)
- ✓ Pediatric and Preventive Dentistry
  (Paedodontist)
- ✓ Conservative and Endodontic Dentistry
  (Endodontist)
- ✓ Oral and Maxillofacial Surgery
  (Oral Surgeon)
- ✓ Periodontology
  (Periodontist)
- ✓ Oral and Maxillofacial Pathology
  (Oral Pathologist)
- ✓ Public Health Dentistry

> **Good Oral Health = Good Overall Health**

Principles of Ethics

- Do not harm.
- Justice.
- To do good.
- Truthfulness.
- Confidentiality.
- Respect for autonomy (informed consent).

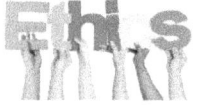

Oral hygiene is preventive care. This means you can stop oral health problems such as cavities, gum disease, bad breath and other issues before they start by taking good care of your teeth and gums.

Dental council of India

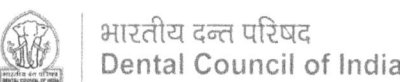
भारतीय दन्त परिषद
Dental Council of India

- The Dentist Act was established in 1948, under which the Dental Council of India was established on 12 April 1949 the purpose of which was to regulate the Dental education and the Profession of Dentistry throughout India.
- The Dental council provides recognition to various colleges in India, after the fulfilment of predetermined criteria and allows the following courses for dental education.

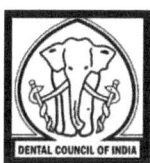

- B.D.S. (Bachelor of Dental Surgery)
- M.D.S. (Master in Dental Surgery)
- Dental Hygienist
- Dental Mechanics

DCI framed a code of ethics in 1975, the goal of which is to treat dentists, staff members, and all patients with dignity and respect.

> **Teeth Are Precious Treat Them Like It.**

Origin

Pierre Fauchard (1678 -1761)

FATHER of Modern Dentistry –

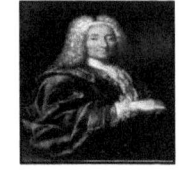

He is a distinguished observer and recorder of dental disease and was one of the first people to stress the importance of oral hygiene.

Dr. Rafiuddin Ahmed

FATHER of Dentistry in India-

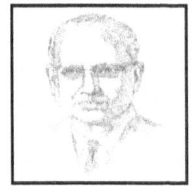

Dr. Rafiuddin Ahmed (24 December 1890 – 9 February 1965) was an Indian dentist, educator, and later minister in the West Bengal cabinet, who founded the first dental college of India, **Dr. R. Ahmed Dental College and Hospital,** later named 'The Calcutta Dental College', where he remained its principal until 1950.

> Indian Dental Association declared **24 December** as National Dentist Day.

Important Days

January	22	- Prosthodontist Day
February	04	- World Cancer Day
	13	– Oral and Maxillofacial Day
	23	- National Periodontist Day
	25	- National Oral Pathologist Day
	28	- National Tooth Fairy Day
March	05	- Conservative and Endodontic Day
	20	- World Oral Health Day
April		Oral Cancer Awareness Month
	07	- World Health Day
May	12	-Gum Health Day
	15	-World Orthodontic Health Day
	31	-No Tobacco Day
June		Oral Health Month
	19-	Public Health Dentistry Day
July	1	-Doctors Day
	27	- Head and Neck Cancer Day
October	1	-International Day of Elderly
November	07	- Toothbrush Day
	10	-World Radiology Day

Don't Wait Unti You Loose All.

Anatomy of Tooth

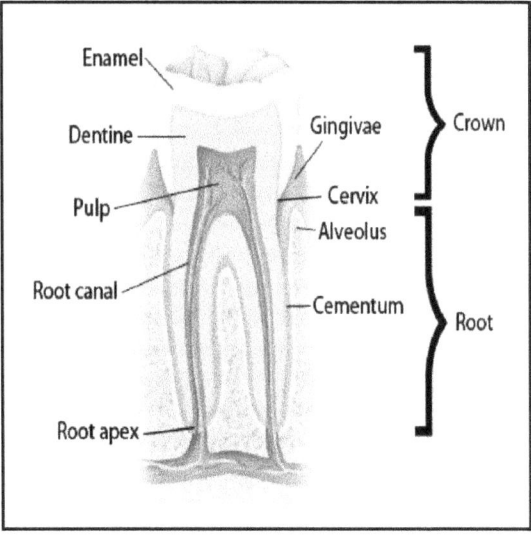

General tooth anatomy indicates the four primary types of dental tissue: enamel, dentine, pulp, and cementum. Adapted from Nanci, 2003.

Teeth Is The Only Part Of The Body Which Cannot Be Healed By Itself So Take Care Of It.

Different Parts of a Tooth

- **Crown** — the top part of the tooth, and the only part you can normally see. The shape of the crown determines the tooth's function. For example, front teeth are sharp and chisel-shaped for cutting, while molars have flat surfaces for grinding.
- **Gumline** — where the tooth and the gums meet. Without proper brushing and flossing, plaque and tartar can build up at the gum line, leading to gingivitis and gum disease.
- **Root** — the part of the tooth that is embedded in bone. The root makes up about two-thirds of the tooth and holds the tooth in place.
- **Enamel** — the outermost layer of the tooth. Enamel is the hardest, most mineralized tissue in the body — yet it can be damaged by decay if teeth are not cared for properly.
- **Dentin** — the layer of the tooth under the enamel. If decay is able to progress its way through the enamel, it next attacks the dentin — where millions of tiny tubes lead directly to the dental pulp.
- **Pulp** — the soft tissue found in the center of all teeth, where the nerve tissue and blood vessels are. If tooth decay reaches the pulp, you usually feel pain.

> **Smile Today and Always**

Different Types of Teeth?

Every tooth has a specific job or function (use the dental arch in this section to locate and identify each type of tooth):

- **Incisors** — the sharp, chisel-shaped front teeth (four upper, four lower) used for cutting food.

- **Canines** — sometimes called cuspids, these teeth are shaped like points (cusps) and are used for tearing food.

- **Premolars** — these teeth have two pointed cusps on their biting surface and are sometimes referred to as bicuspids. The premolars are for crushing and tearing.

- **Molars** — used for grinding, these teeth have several cusps on the biting surface.

> **Brushing Harder Does Not Clean Better.**

Dentition

Natural teeth in position in the dental arches.

1. Primary Dentition (Deciduous Dentition)

The number of teeth present in the child is usually 20 if none are congenitally missing or lost as a result of disease.

The eruption is expected to begin at 6 months of age.

Usually at age 2 to 2.5 years or thereabout, primary dentition is completed.

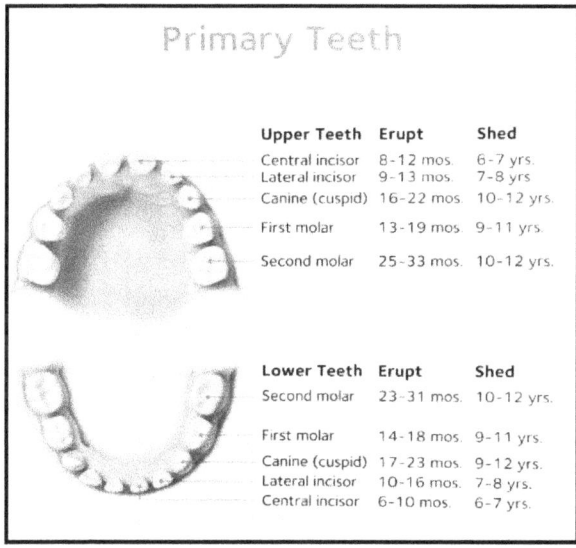

Upper Teeth	Erupt	Shed
Central incisor	8-12 mos.	6-7 yrs.
Lateral incisor	9-13 mos.	7-8 yrs.
Canine (cuspid)	16-22 mos.	10-12 yrs.
First molar	13-19 mos.	9-11 yrs.
Second molar	25-33 mos.	10-12 yrs.

Lower Teeth	Erupt	Shed
Second molar	23-31 mos.	10-12 yrs.
First molar	14-18 mos.	9-11 yrs.
Canine (cuspid)	17-23 mos.	9-12 yrs.
Lateral incisor	10-16 mos.	7-8 yrs.
Central incisor	6-10 mos.	6-7 yrs.

> **One Of The Strongest Muscle In The Human Body Is The Tongue.**

2. **MIXED DENTITION**- usually exists from 6 to 12 years of age. This is the combination of primary and permanent teeth. It occurs as the permanent teeth begin to erupt within the oral cavity, while some of the primary teeth are still present.

3. **PERMANENT DENTITION**- 32 teeth of adulthood. The eruption is expected to begin at 6 years of age. Usually, at age 17 to 21 years, the permanent dentition is completed.

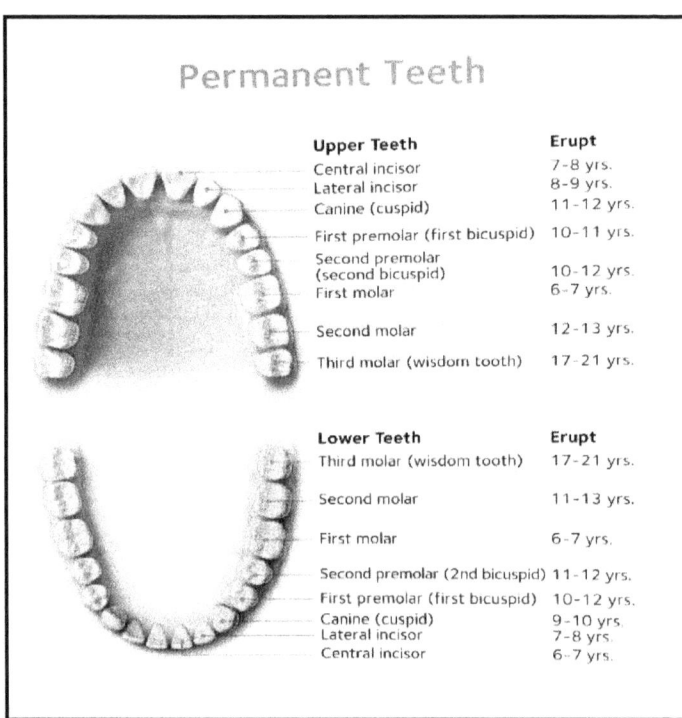

Permanent Teeth

Upper Teeth	Erupt
Central incisor	7-8 yrs.
Lateral incisor	8-9 yrs.
Canine (cuspid)	11-12 yrs.
First premolar (first bicuspid)	10-11 yrs.
Second premolar (second bicuspid)	10-12 yrs.
First molar	6-7 yrs.
Second molar	12-13 yrs.
Third molar (wisdom tooth)	17-21 yrs.

Lower Teeth	Erupt
Third molar (wisdom tooth)	17-21 yrs.
Second molar	11-13 yrs.
First molar	6-7 yrs.
Second premolar (2nd bicuspid)	11-12 yrs.
First premolar (first bicuspid)	10-12 yrs.
Canine (cuspid)	9-10 yrs.
Lateral incisor	7-8 yrs.
Central incisor	6-7 yrs.

Shark's Teeth Are as Hard as Steel.

Primary Dentition V/S Permanent Dentition

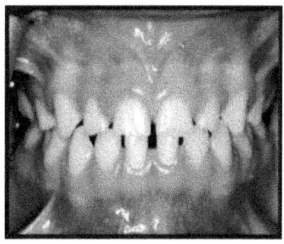 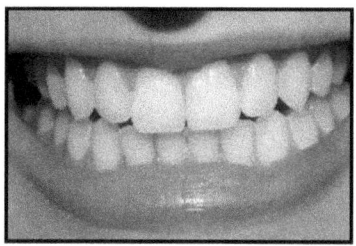

- Consists of 20 teeth (10 in each arch)
- Begins to erupt around the 6th month of post-natal life and continues till the 13th month of post-natal life
- Teeth are smaller in size with space (generalized and primate) between the teeth
- Shedding being at around 6 years of age

- Consists of 32 teeth (16 in each arch)
- Eruption begins at 6 years of age and lasts till 12 years of age and the #rd molar erupts between 18 – 25 years of age
- This does not undergo physiologic shedding, however loosening and subsequent exfoliation may occur due to pathologic conditions

Smile, It Lets Your Teeth Breathe.

Functions of the Tooth and the Oral Cavity

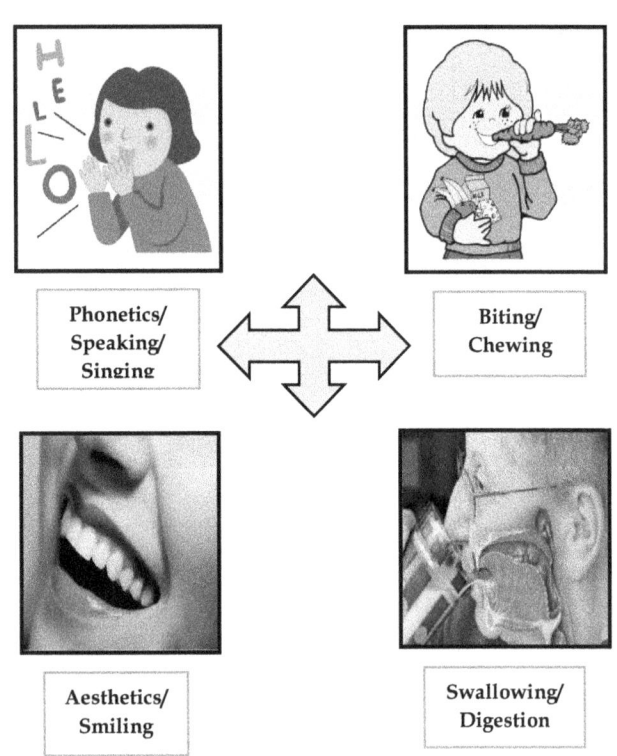

- Phonetics/ Speaking/ Singing
- Biting/ Chewing
- Aesthetics/ Smiling
- Swallowing/ Digestion

If You Don't Floss, You Miss Cleaning 40% Of Your Tooth Surfaces, Make Sure You Brush And Floss Twice A Day.

Tips for Better Dental Health

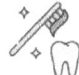 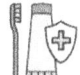 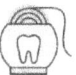

BRUSH TEETH REGULARLY   USE A FLUORIDE TOOTHPASTE   FLOSS ONCE A DAY   SEE A DENTIST REGULARLY

TIPS FOR BETTER DENTAL HEALTH

   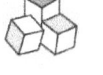

CONSIDER A MOUTHWASH   DO NOT SMOKE   LIMIT SUGARY FOODS   DRINK MORE WATER

Who Invented First Tooth Brush?

William Addis of Clerkenwald, England Around 1780

Dos and Don'ts

Dos	Don'ts
✓ High fibrous diet	✗ Diet with high sugar content
✓ Diet rich in vitamins and antioxidants	✗ Excessive intake of acidic drinks
✓ Meticulous brushing twice daily	✗ Smoking
✓ Rinsing of mouth after every meal	✗ Alcohol
✓ Regular visit to the dentist (every 3 – 6 months)	✗ Tobacco use
	✗ Poor oral hygiene

Investing In Your Smile Is Always A Worthwhile.

What problems could Poor Dental Health Cause

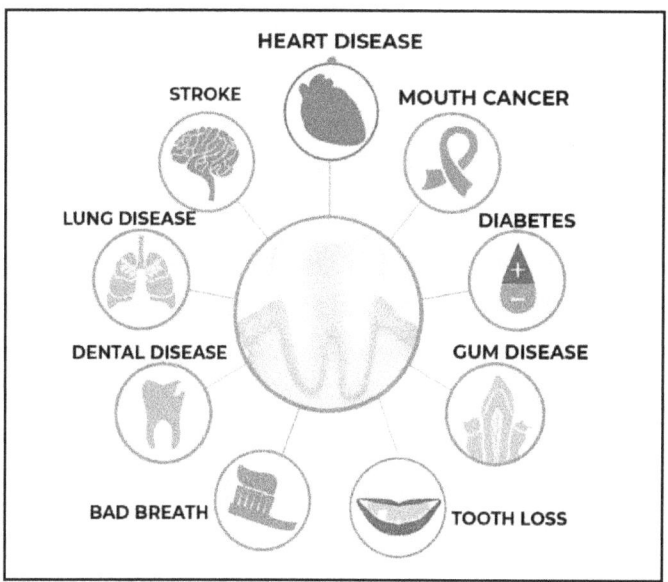

Tongue Plays An Important Role In Reducing Bad Breath.

Don't Forget To Clean Your Tongue Daily.

Do You Feel Nervous about the Dentist?

Phobia vs. Anxiety

Suppose you feel some nervousness or stress before a dental appointment. In that case, you are grappling with a type of anxiety that is relatively common. But someone with a dental phobia has such intense fear, just the thought of going to the dentist can cause them to panic. Those with dental phobia are encouraged to seek professional help from licensed therapists or counselors for coping mechanisms before their appointment.

Causes of Fear

Someone with an intense fear of the dentist is usually reacting to memories of an unpleasant experience in the past, whether it's the result of a painful incident or a similarly upsetting life event. Those who experience mild anxiety before a dental appointment; on the other hand, may just be nervous about a procedure they have yet to experience. Still, others equate a dental visit with pain because their prior experience wasn't as pleasant as today's pain-free dentistry allows.

> Like Fingerprints, Everyone's Tongue Print Is Different.

Facing It

If you haven't been to a dentist for over a year because of fear, your teeth and gums may be paying the price. The good news is dentists today understand these fears and are doing what they can to make dental appointments more comfortable for their patients. For example, dental offices now take on friendlier environments than in the past, with cozy waiting rooms, soothing music, and staff who know how to make the appointment feel less like a formal event. So don't be embarrassed to discuss your concerns and fears with your dentist. Together you can customize solutions to reduce your stress level during future treatment.

Your dentist may ease you into dental treatment by scheduling simple procedures like exams or cleaning before starting more complicated procedures. They may even suggest some form of anaesthesia or sedation to eliminate pain and anxiety during this treatment stage. Dentists often use distraction to calm fears, too – headphones for music or goggles for watching videos, both of which can divert your attention away from the process itself. Of course, nervous patients should consider using their own relaxation techniques as well.

> **Dogs Have 42 Teeth.**
> **Pigs Have 44 Teeth.**
> **Armadillos Have 104 Teeth.**

Tips for Easing Dental Fears

1. Ask friends and family- If you don't already have a dentist, ask people you trust about their dentist and be happy with their provider. Word of mouth is a great way to find a good dentist.

2. Search for a dentist online- Many dental offices have websites where you can learn about their practices and become familiar with the staff. If you have found a few dental practices that look promising, ask friends and neighbours about them and visit once.

3. Talk about your feelings- Once you choose a dentist, make sure you communicate with the dentist and staff. Don't be shy! You are not the first patient who ever felt nervous or anxious. Talking will make your dental experience more relaxed and pleasant.

4. Ask questions- Ask your dental team to inform you about the type of dental treatment they recommend based on your unique oral health needs. Once a treatment plan has been developed, ask your dentist to explain the procedures in detail. Knowing what to expect before it happens can help put your mind at ease.

5. Try to relax- If you are nervous before going to a professional cleaning or dental procedure, talk to the dentist about making the experience more comfortable. The dentist and staff should make every effort to make your visit comforting and less stressful.

> **Giraffes Only Have Bottom Teeth.**

Overcoming Fear with Prevention

Regular dental check-ups and cleanings are always essential to keep your mouth healthy. But it's the oral care at home that can keep you from needing more complicated dental procedures down the line. Whether or not you have a fear of the dentist, brush your teeth thoroughly twice a day with fluoride toothpaste, floss at least once daily, and limit sugary snacks between your main courses.

As you and your dentist work to make your visits more relaxed, it won't take long for fears and stress to start to weaken. And as each dental appointment becomes more comfortable, your teeth and gums will become healthier and your smile more confident.

> **Even Babies Are Prone To Cavities.**

Habits That Ruin Your Teeth

1. Utilizing Your Teeth as a Tool

We use our teeth for consuming food, but we often end up using them as our primary tool for several activities. We often use our teeth to open a bottle, bite nails, chew ice etc. But these activities can cause damage to the teeth and should be avoided.

2. Biting Your Nails

Biting the nails is one of the most common habits that is found these days and this is a habit that can prove harmful to your teeth in the long run. It can very much damage the shape of your teeth and once it starts affecting your teeth, you will start experiencing severe teeth pain. Its best to avoid such a bad habit and make sure that your teeth remain healthy and strong.

3. Use of Tobacco

Tobacco is one of the deadliest habits. Tobacco use has a lot of serious health issues and most of these issues are life threatening. The use of tobacco will also make sure that you have gum problems on a regular basis, which will also damage your teeth. So, stay away from tobacco for a better health, teeth and smile.

> **It Is Safe to Visit Dentist During Pregnancy.**

4. Chewing of Ice

Chewing of ice seems harmless, but the irony is that chewing of ice is not a good habit for your throat, as well as your teeth. Your teeth and its roots will always stand a chance of getting damaged by the regular chewing of ice. You might get some pleasure while chewing the ice, but at the same time you are risking the health of your teeth.

5. Usage of Toothpicks in an Incorrect Way

Whenever we eat certain type of food materials, especially chicken or meat, a lot of the good residue will get stuck in the gaps of our teeth. This will be distracting for us and hence we will seek the help of tooth picks to get rid of those food materials from our teeth. If you are not using the tooth pick in the proper way, then you are certainly going to damage your gum and teeth in a bad way.

6. Consuming Too Much Sugary Foods and Beverages

We all love sugary foods and beverages and at times we cannot resist ourselves from having such food items. Sugary foods and beverages might taste good, but it is very much harmful to our teeth and damages our teeth drastically. A continuous consumption of sugary foods and beverages might damage your teeth causing gum infection and toothache.

7. Not Brushing Your Teeth Regularly

Brushing our teeth is one of the most basic actions that lead to a better and healthy tooth. Majority of the people make sure to brush at least twice in a day to make their teeth shine better and remain healthy. If you are not brushing your teeth regularly, you will be risking the health of your teeth and the chances of it getting decayed becomes higher.

8. Grinding Your Teeth

Some of us have the habit of grinding our teeth even while asleep and this is something that can take a toll on the enamel, leading to other dental health problems. So, if you are serious about the health of your teeth, then it is better to make sure that you avoid the habit of grinding your teeth.

9. Using a Tooth-Brush That Has Hard Bristles

Tooth-brushes are an essential part of maintaining the cleanliness of our teeth and hence it is something that we cannot compromise upon. Most of the time we might be using a toothbrush having hard bristles, which are very much harmful to our gums. Always make sure that you use a toothbrush that have soft bristles and do not damage the gums in any ways.

10. Regular Use of Soda

Soda or Pop, is a drink that we often consume to get rid of our thirst. It is fine to drink soda once in a while, but if it becomes a regular habit, it can become harmful to your tooth. Soda can easily damage the enamel and make your teeth weak and infected in the long run. So better stay away from soda and other carbonated drink whenever possible.

The above tips can be very much beneficial for maintaining the overall health of your teeth and remember that once you start losing your teeth, life will not be the same again even though you can compensate it through various implants.

> **Broken Teeth Can Be Saved.**

11. Tongue thrusting

Pushing teeth with tongue can result into misalignment of teeth and causing duck like appearance.

12. Thumb sucking

Thumb sucking isn't usually a concern until a child's permanent teeth come in. At this point, thumb sucking might begin to affect the roof of the mouth (palate) or how the teeth line up. The risk of dental problems is related to how often, how long and how intensely your child sucks on his or her thumb.

13. Mouth breathing

Mouth breathing can cause sleep disorders that affect daily life. It can also change the structure of people's faces. Most people develop mouth breathing as very young children, potentially setting the stage for long-term problems.

Choose Water Over Sugary Drinks.

How Often Should You Visit the Dentist?

While it's true that visiting the dentist twice a year is a good rule of thumb for many people, the truth is that you have your own unique smile needs. So, it depends on your oral hygiene, habits, and individual medical conditions.

Some people only need to visit the dentist once or twice are year, while others may need to go more often. So, always remember to ask your dentist when you should schedule your next appointment. And don't worry! They'll probably tell you when they want to see you next anyway.

Better Teeth Better Health.

Who Should Go to the Dentist More Often?

Some people need to visit the dentist more than twice a year. But who? People with a greater risk of dental disease and other health conditions may need to see the dentist every three months or more. This higher-risk group includes:

- Pregnant women.
- Smokers.
- Diabetics.
- People with gum disease.
- People with a weak immune response.
- People who are prone to cavities or plaque build-up.

> To protect your oral health, practice good oral hygiene daily.

Why is Going to the Dentist Important?

Even if you brush twice a day and floss daily, you still need to visit a dentist regularly! Your dentist and dental hygienist are trained to check for problems that you might not see or feel on your own. Some things, like cavities or gum disease, aren't even visible or painful until they're more advanced. When it comes to oral cancer, the Indian Dental Association suggests that your dentist can diagnose early signs of oral cancer.

Because the issue might either be preventable or more easily treated when caught early (like oral cancer), seeing a dentist regularly matters. With regular visits, your dentist will find solutions to any red flags that will save you time, discomfort, and even money in the long run.

Don't Rush When You Brush.

What Can You Do to Keep Dentist Appointments to a Minimum?

The best thing you can do to keep your dental visits to a minimum is to maintain good oral hygiene. So, make sure to brush your teeth twice a day and clean between your teeth daily using floss, interdental brushes, or an oral irrigator. And guess what? If your dentist doesn't see any cavities or signs of gingivitis for several years, they might even lengthen the time between your visits.

Now you know that how often you need to visit the dentist depends on your unique smile situation. For some people, like smokers and diabetics, it may be more often. But no matter what, visiting the dentist is a preventative measure that improves your overall health and makes things easier for you in the long run. If you keep up with your daily hygiene, your dentist may even cut back on your required dental appointments. Remember to always follow your dentist's advice in terms of your next appointment. And if it's been a while, it's time to respond to that text, call, or email from your dentist office for your 6-month dental check-in.

> **Clean Between Your Teeth Daily Using Floss, Or Interdental Brushes.**

Oral Health for Diabetics

Diabetes is a disease on the rise, particularly among children and adolescents. Apart from the serious health problems caused by this condition, there can often be complications you might not expect — and they spell bad news for your gums and teeth. Here's what to look out for.

Gum problems

This is one of the most common complaints of diabetes sufferers. In fact, people with diabetes are two times more likely to develop gum disease which leads to the advanced stage known as periodontitis. As their condition makes them more prone to infections, diabetics are at risk from germs that attack their gums.

Dry mouth

Because of the medications they take, people with diabetes may have to endure the side effect of dry mouth. This lack of saliva can lead to other problems such as infections — without saliva, you're more likely to get a cavity, as there is very little liquid to wash away germs. Be sure to drink plenty of water to maintain a moist mouth.

Did You Know?

According to the International Diabetes Federation, there were 61.3 million people in India with diabetes in 2011. As this figure continues to rise, India has the second highest rate of people living with diabetes in the world, just behind China.

A two-way street

Unfortunately, not only can diabetes cause gum problems, but gum problems can also worsen uncontrolled diabetes. Once it reaches a certain stage, gum disease can start to affect your blood glucose level, hastening the onset of diabetes or worsening the condition. During each visit, it is important to communicate with your medical doctor and dentist about your oral health and state of diabetes control.

Keep your eyes open

Gum disease does not always make itself known through pain. Chronic gum problems are painless, so you have to be vigilant and visit the dentist for regular check-ups. Kids, in particular, may not know what to look out for, so if you notice they have swollen gums, or are bleeding after they brush their teeth, visit a dentist immediately. Loosened teeth or a persistent bad taste in the mouth are also symptoms.

Prevention is the cure

The prevention or control of diabetes is down to making smart lifestyle choices. Eating a healthy diet is important, as is regular exercise 30 minutes a day.

Care For Your Smile.

If you are a person living with and managing diabetes, good healthcare for you goes beyond just balancing the blood sugar; taking care of your mouth and gums is also an important goal. One oral health problem to keep an eye out for is an infection of the tissues that support your teeth called gum disease. But, just spending that extra moment to care for your mouth and gums can go a long way in avoiding gum disease, which can aid in better diabetes management.

What are the early signs?

According to the American Dental Association, there are several preludes to this condition, such as:

- Bleeding and swollen gums
- Bad breath
- Any change in the way your teeth fit together when you bite

Keeping gums healthy, with just a little bit of extra care

The good news is, preventing and even taking care of early-stage gum disease is easy! The Dentist suggests the following best practices to adopt to keep it away:

- Time yourself: Brushing your teeth and gum line for two minutes twice a day is a good rule of thumb. Use a soft bristle brush, unless indicated otherwise by your dentist.

An Elephant Tooth Can Weight Over 6 Pounds.

- Floss right: If you ask any dentist the one key oral hygiene practice, which people tend to skip, it's flossing. Floss every day carefully between each tooth but do it gently by sliding the floss up and down and back and forth to avoid bleeding.
- Remember the tongue: The bacteria find a home in the tongue too, so remember to also gently brush your tongue for a few seconds as a part of your routine. Antimicrobial mouthwashes and tongue cleaners can also help here.
- Eat well: Avoid acidic drinks, which can erode the tooth enamel and may lead to decay. Studies also show that certain diets may help reduce the chances of gum disease, so consult your dentist about what to eat.
- See the experts: Lastly, visit your dentist or hygienist at least once a year even if you have healthy gums, and if you've noticed any of the warning signs, be sure to report it.

Avoid Sticky and Acidic Foods

Oral Medicine & Radiology

What does an ORAL RADIOLOGIST do?

Dental specialization that deals with the diagnosis of oral diseases, oral manifestations of systemic diseases, and dental treatment of medically compromised patients.

It is the department of diagnosis.

It compiles of-

1) Case history

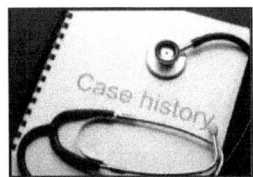

2) oral examination and diagnosis

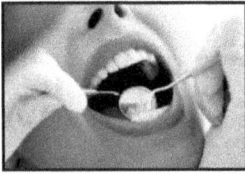

3) TMJ Examination

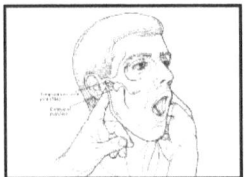

4) Public awareness

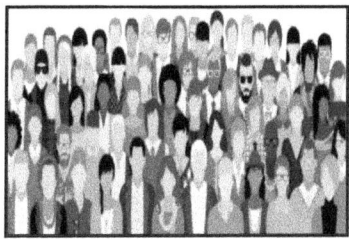

5) Diagnostic instruments are tweezers, probes, and mouth mirrors.

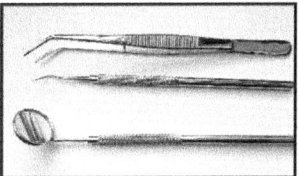

> **Limit Sugar Intake to Avoid Decay.**

Supportive Investigations

Teeth are like icebergs in the sea, we can see only 30% of them with the naked eye, and need investigating X-rays to view them at fuller

William C. Rontgen- Father of Diagnostic Radiology
Dr. C. Edmund Kells – Father of Dental Radiology

> **A Tooth's Natural Color Is Slightly Yellowish.**

Why Dental X-Rays Are Performed

Dental radiographs can alert your dentist to changes in your hard and soft tissues. In children, radiographs allow the dentist to see how their teeth and jawbones are developing. Like medical radiographs, dental radiographs allow your dentist to evaluate any injuries to your face and mouth.

In addition to its preventive care purposes, an X-ray is also a helpful tool for planning a course of treatment for patients who are having restorative care, dental implants placed, or other cosmetic care.

Common Dental Radiography

1- Intraoral X-Ray

INTRA ORAL PERIAPICAL RADIOGRAPH (IOPAR)

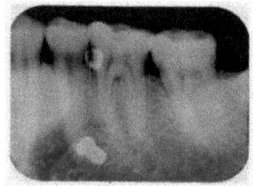

- Most common Dental Xray
- Easier
- Cheaper
- Comfortable for the patient
- Covers 2-3 teeth
- **DOSE-:** 0.005mSv(millisieverts)

Indications-:

- Development of the root end, unerupted tooth, and periapical tissues.
- Deep dental caries, small cyst associated with tooth
- The prognosis of the Pulp treatment (Root canal treatment).
- Developmental abnormalities like Supernumerary, missing or malformed teeth.

RVG (Radio Visio Graphy)

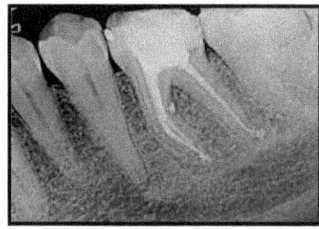

- It is the latest advancement in dental imaging.

Indications-:

- With minimal radiation exposure to the patient.
- Detection of tumors.
- Detection of metastatic hard tissue lesions.
- Detection of caries and periodontal tissues.
- Detection of any perforation to the surrounding soft tissue (e.g. Maxillary sinus).

> Coconuts are natural anti-bacterial food and can help reduce the risk of developing gum diseases and cavities

2-Extraoral X-Ray

OPG (Orthopantomogram)-

- For a complete and wider view of the jaw at once.
- Display all the teeth on both jaws on one film, including those that have not surfaced or erupted yet, such as wisdom teeth

DOSE-: 7mSv

Indications-:

- Evaluation of trauma (Fracture)
- Third molars
- Large lesions
- Tooth development
- Developmental anomalies
- Intolerant to intraoral procedures.

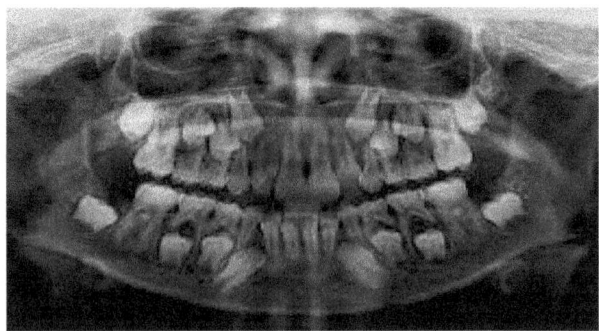

> Don't Go To The Bed Without Brushing Your Teeth.

CBCT (Cone Beam Computed Tomography)

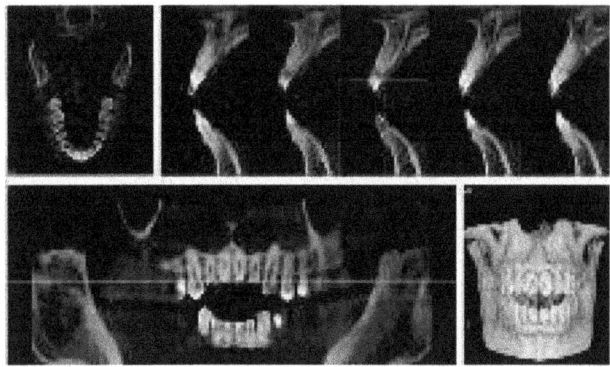

It is a radiographic imaging method that allows accurate three-dimensional (3D) Imaging of hard tissue structures.

DOSE: 12mSv(millisieverts)

Indications-:

Provide detailed 3D images of the Facial bone and are performed to evaluate Any kind of deformity, obstruction, fracture, and lesion of the Face, ear, nose, and throat.

> **Your Smile Is Beautiful Don't Stain With Nicotine.**

Few Common Lesions

Oral candidiasis (Thrush).

Candidiasis is a fungal infection caused by an overgrowth of a type of yeast that lives on your body (Candida albicans). A candidiasis infection often appears on your skin, vagina, or mouth, where Candida naturally lives in small amounts. Healthy bacteria in your body prevent yeast overgrowth. Imagine you have a two-armed scale with healthy bacteria on one side and yeast on the other. The scale stays balanced until disruption occurs from stress, a poor diet, a weakened immune system, or an uncontrolled medical condition. When something disrupts your scale, a Candidiasis infection occurs.

Whom does candidiasis affect?

- People with diabetes.
- People who are pregnant.
- Babies and infants.
- People who wear dentures.
- Hospitalized individuals.
- People with poor oral hygiene.

> **Tooth Pulp Is Vital in Keeping the Tooth Healthy. It Is Considered To Be The Heart Of The Tooth.**

How does candidiasis affect your body?

Candidiasis causes discomfort, itching, and irritation until you find treatment, but is not a major threat to your overall health. Like any other infection that you might get from an injury, it's best to treat the infection at the first sign to alleviate your symptoms. If candidiasis is left untreated, severe infections could spread to other parts of your body, including your blood, heart, and brain.

Symptoms And Causes

What are the symptoms of candidiasis?

Symptoms of candidiasis vary depending on the location of the infection. Symptoms of candidiasis include:

- Itching.
- Burning sensation.
- Scrapable white patches or sores in your mouth that cause loss of taste or pain when eating or swallowing.
- Swelling (inflammation).

What causes candidiasis?

A candidiasis infection is the result of an overgrowth of Candida yeast due to an imbalance of healthy bacteria and yeast in your body. Triggers that disrupt the balance of bacteria and yeast include:

- Taking antibiotics, steroids, oral contraceptives, medicines that cause dry mouth, or medicines that turn off healthy bacteria.
- Feeling stressed.

- Eating a diet high in refined carbohydrates, sugar, or yeast.
- Having uncontrolled diabetes, HIV, cancer, or a compromised immune system.
- Experiencing hormonal changes (pregnancy).

Is candidiasis contagious?

Candida yeast can spread from person to person, but that doesn't mean it's contagious like the flu virus. If you come in contact with someone who has candidiasis, you won't necessarily develop the infection because the yeast on another person didn't change the balance of yeast and bacteria in your body, but it's a possibility that it could change your balance, and cause an infection.

For parents who are chest feeding (breastfeeding) a newborn, if your child acquires oral candidiasis (thrush), that infection can transfer to you via your baby's saliva. If this occurs, your healthcare provider will recommend treatment for both you and your baby's infections at the same time to prevent the infections from coming back.

How is candidiasis diagnosed?

Your healthcare provider will diagnose candidiasis after a **physical examination** of the affected area. They will also ask you questions about your symptoms, including the severity of your symptoms and how long you've experienced them. Your healthcare provider will also test the infection to identify the type of yeast that is overgrown, which better determines your treatment options.

What tests help diagnose candidiasis?

Your healthcare provider will test the infection to determine the best treatment plan to combat the overgrowth of yeast. A **culture test** identifies the type of yeast and bacteria in your infection. For this test, your healthcare provider will swab the infected area with sterile cotton, then examine the sample under a microscope.

If your healthcare provider suspects invasive candidiasis, they may draw a sample of your blood to examine whether or not yeast and bacteria spread into your bloodstream.

How do I get rid of candidiasis?

After diagnosis, your healthcare provider will recommend several different treatment options depending on the type of candidiasis you have. All candidiasis treatment involves using or taking **an antifungal medication that is either oral (pill, lozenge, or liquid**) or topical (cream or ointment). Each antifungal medicine has specific instructions, so make sure you ask your healthcare provider to explain how to apply or take the medication and how long you should take it.

Even if your symptoms stop early, it's best to continue your treatment plan as advised by your healthcare provider to eliminate the infection and prevent it from returning.

How long does candidiasis last?

Most mild to moderate cases of candidiasis will clear up **in two to three days** after your complete treatment. More severe cases of candidiasis may take a couple of weeks to clear up completely after treatment.

How can I prevent candidiasis?

You can prevent candidiasis by:

- Maintaining good physical and oral hygiene.
- Minimizing unhealthy foods from your diet like refined carbohydrates and sugar.
- Managing your stress.
- Treating current medical conditions like diabetes, cancer or HIV.
- Talk with your healthcare provider about current medications you are taking that might cause candidiasis as a side effect.

What can I expect if I have candidiasis?

Treatment for candidiasis is extremely effective. Symptoms are bothersome but will start to fade after treatment begins and infections will clear up completely between two to three days or up to two weeks, depending on the type and severity of infection. If left untreated, symptoms of candidiasis will cause irritation and discomfort and could increase in severity over time. Sometimes candidiasis will return after treatment, so it's best to work with your healthcare provider on a treatment plan to target the specific type of yeast that caused the overgrowth on your body and follow through on treatment as directed.

LEUKOPLAKIA- What is leukoplakia?

Leukoplakia are one or more white patches on the surface of the tongue, underneath the tongue, or on the insides of the cheeks. The patches cannot be rubbed off and cannot be traced to any other cause. No pain or other symptoms are present.

What are the causes of leukoplakia?

Leukoplakia is often associated with the following:

- Heavy smoking.
- Use of chewing tobacco or snuff
- Chewing areca nut (also known as betel nut), which grows in the tropics of Asia, the Pacific, and parts of East Africa.
- Heavy use of alcohol (although not all studies show this link).

How is leukoplakia diagnosed?

Since the white patches of leukoplakia do not cause symptoms, they are often first noticed by healthcare providers during a routine examination.

Before a diagnosis of leukoplakia is made, other possible causes of the white patches are investigated. These could include friction inside the mouth (caused by something such as dentures), repeated biting of the cheek, fungal infection or lichen planus.

If no cause is found and the white patches are not gone after two to four weeks, a biopsy (tissue sample) is taken and sent to the laboratory for examination.

If the biopsy still does not show a clear diagnosis, the white patch may be confirmed as leukoplakia, meaning that it has the potential to become cancerous. (If cancer cells are actually found, this means a diagnosis of cancer, not of leukoplakia.)

What is the prognosis (outlook) for patients who have leukoplakia?

Anyone who has leukoplakia should follow up with a doctor every three to six months, with biopsies as needed, to watch for possible changes in the condition.

Even if patches are surgically removed, an examination every six to 12 months is recommended, because leukoplakia frequently returns. Treatment sites that remain free of abnormalities for three years may not need to be observed anymore.

OSMF Oral submucous fibrosis.

Oral submucous fibrosis (OSF) is a premalignant condition caused by betel chewing. It is very common in Southeast Asia but has started to spread to Europe and North America. OSF can lead to squamous cell carcinoma, a risk that is further increased by concomitant tobacco consumption. OSF is a diagnosis based on clinical symptoms and confirmation by histopathology. Hypo vascularity leading to blanching of the oral mucosa, staining of teeth and gingiva, and trismus are major symptoms.

> Take Care of Your Teeth and They Will Take Care of You.

Symptoms-

In the initial phase of the disease, the mucosa feels leathery with palpable fibrotic bands. In the advanced stage, the oral mucosa loses its resiliency and becomes blanched and stiff. The disease is believed to begin in the posterior part of the oral cavity and gradually spread outward.

Other features of the disease include:

- Xerostomia
- Recurrent ulceration
- Pain in the ear or deafness
- Nasal intonation of voice
- Restriction of the movement of the soft palate
- A budlike shrunken uvula.
- Thinning and stiffening of the lips
- Pigmentation of the oral mucosa
- Dryness of the mouth and burning sensation (stomatopyrosis).
- Decreased mouth opening and tongue protrusion.

Causes-

Dried products such as paan masala and gutka have higher concentrations of areca nut and appear to cause the disease. Other causes include:

- Immunological diseases
- Extreme climatic conditions
- Prolonged deficiency of iron and vitamins in the diet

Diagnosis

Classification

Oral submucous fibrosis is clinically divided into three stages:

- Stage 1: Stomatitis
- Stage 2: Fibrosis

  a- Early lesions, blanching of the oral mucosa

  b- Older lesions, vertical and circular palpable fibrous bands in and around the mouth or lips, resulting in a mottled, marble-like appearance of the buccal mucosa

- Stage 3: Sequelae of oral submucous fibrosis

  a- leukoplakia

  b- Speech and hearing deficits

Treatment

Biopsy screening although necessary is not mandatory most dentists can visually examine the area and proceed with the proper course of treatment.

Treatment includes:

- Abstention from chewing areca nut (also known as betel nut) and tobacco
- Minimizing consumption of spicy foods, including chiles
- Maintaining proper oral hygiene
- Supplementing the diet with foods rich in vitamins A, B complex, and C and iron
- Forgoing hot fluids like tea, coffee

- Forgoing alcohol
- Employing a dental surgeon to round off sharp teeth and extract third molars
- Interprofessional treatment approach

Treatment also includes the following:

- The prescription of chewable pellets of hydrocortisone (Efcorlin); one pellet to be chewed every three to four hours for three to four weeks
- 0.5 ml intralesional injection of Hyaluronidase 1500 IU mixed in 1 ml of Lignocaine into each buccal mucosa once a week for 4 weeks or more as per condition
- 0.5 ml intralesional injection of Hyaluronidase 1500 IU and 0.5 ml of injection of Hydrocortisone acetate 25 mg/ml in each buccal mucosa once a week alternatively for 4 weeks or more as per condition
- Submucosal injections of hydrocortisone 100 mg once or twice daily depending upon the severity of the disease for two to three weeks
- Submucosal injections of human chorionic gonadotrophins (Placentrax) 2-3 ml per sitting twice or thrice a week for three to four weeks
- Surgical treatment is recommended in cases of progressive fibrosis when the inter-incisor distance becomes less than 2 centimeters (0.79 in). (Multiple release incisions deep to the mucosa, submucosa, and fibrotic tissue and suturing the gap or dehiscence so created by mucosal graft obtained

The treatment of patients with oral submucous fibrosis depends on the degree of clinical involvement. If the disease is detected at a very early stage, cessation of the habit is sufficient. Most patients with oral submucous fibrosis present with moderate-to-severe disease. Severe oral submucous fibrosis is irreversible. Moderate oral submucous fibrosis is reversible with cessation of habit and mouth-opening exercise. Current modern-day medical treatments can make the mouth open to normal minimum levels of 30 mm mouth-opening with proper treatment.

Oral Cancer

Oral cancer includes cancers of the mouth and the back of the throat. Oral cancers develop on the tongue, the tissue lining the mouth and gums, under the tongue, at the base of the tongue, and the area of the throat at the back of the mouth.

Oral cancer accounts for roughly three percent of all cancers diagnosed annually in the United States, or about 53,000 new cases each year.

Oral cancer most often occurs in people over the age of 40 and affects more than twice as many men as women. Most oral cancers are related to tobacco use, alcohol use (or both), or infection by the human papillomavirus (HPV).

Rinse Between Meals

Causes

Tobacco and alcohol use. Tobacco use of any kind, including cigarette smoking, puts you at risk for developing oral cancers. Heavy alcohol use also increases the risk. Using both tobacco and alcohol increases the risk even further.

HPV. Infection with the sexually transmitted human papillomavirus (specifically the HPV 16 type) has been linked to oral cancers.

Age. Risk increases with age. Oral cancers most often occur in people over the age of 40.

Sun Exposure. Cancer of the lip can be caused by sun exposure.

Symptoms

If you have any of these symptoms for more than two weeks, see a dentist or a doctor.

- A sore, irritation, lump, or thick patch in your mouth, lip, or throat.
- A white or red patch in your mouth.
- A sore throat or a feeling that something is caught in your throat.
- Difficulty chewing, swallowing, or speaking.
- Difficulty moving your jaw or tongue.
- Swelling of your jaw that causes dentures to fit poorly or become uncomfortable.
- Numbness in your tongue or other areas of your mouth.
- Ear pain.

Diagnosis

Because oral cancer can spread quickly, early detection is important. An oral cancer examination can detect early signs of cancer. The exam is painless and takes only a few minutes. Many dentists will perform the test during your regular dental check-up.

During the exam, your dentist or dental hygienist will check your face, neck, lips, and entire mouth for possible signs of cancer.

Treatment

When oral cancer is detected early, it is treated with surgery or radiation therapy. Oral cancer that is further along when it is diagnosed may use a combination of treatments.

For example, radiation therapy and chemotherapy are often given at the same time. Another treatment option is targeted therapy, which is a newer type of cancer treatment that uses drugs or other substances to precisely identify and attack cancer cells. The choice of treatment depends on your general health, where in your mouth or throat the cancer began, the size and type of the tumour, and whether the cancer has spread.

Your doctor may refer you to a specialist. Specialists who treat oral cancer include:

- Head and neck surgeons.
- Dentists who specialize in surgery of the mouth, face, and jaw (oral and maxillofacial surgeons).

> **The First Named Dentist Was An Egyptian Called Hesy-Ra.**

- Ear, nose, and throat doctors (otolaryngologists).
- Doctors who specifically treat cancer (medical and radiation oncologists).

Other health care professionals who may be part of a treatment team include dentists, plastic surgeons, reconstructive surgeons, speech pathologists, oncology nurses, registered dietitians, and mental health counsellors.

What surgeries treat oral cancer?

The most common surgeries for oral cancer are:

- **Primary tumor surgery**: Healthcare providers remove tumors through your mouth or an incision in your neck.
- **Glossectomy**: This is the partial or total removal of your tongue.
- **Mandibulectomy**: This is surgery for oral cancer in your jawbone.
- **Maxillectomy**: This surgery removes part or all of the hard palate, which is the bony roof of your mouth.
- **Sentinel lymph node biopsy**: This test helps healthcare providers know if cancer has spread beyond the original oral cancer.
- **Neck dissection**: This surgery is done to remove lymph nodes from your neck.
- **Reconstruction**: Surgery that removes large areas of tissue might be followed by reconstructive surgery to fill gaps left by the tumor or replace part of your lips, tongue, palate or jaw. In some cases, reconstructive surgery is done by taking healthy bone and tissue from other areas of your body.

What are other ways to treat oral cancer?

Healthcare providers may combine surgery with other treatments, including:

- **Radiation therapy**: Radiation therapy uses strong beams of energy to kill cancer cells or keep them from growing. Your healthcare provider may combine radiation therapy with other treatments.
- **Targeted therapy**: This cancer treatment uses drugs or other substances to precisely identify and attack certain types of cancer cells without hurting normal cells. Monoclonal antibodies are immune system proteins that are created in the lab and used to treat cancer.
- **Chemotherapy**: Your healthcare provider may use anti-cancer drugs that kill cancer cells, including treatments that affect most parts of your body.
- **Immunotherapy**: Immunotherapy is a cancer treatment that engages your immune system to fight the disease.

What can I do to prevent developing oral cancer?

Oral cancer can be prevented, and you can play an active role in preventing it. You can help prevent oral cancer with the following tips:

- If you're someone who smokes tobacco, chews tobacco or uses a water pipe, try stopping or cutting back. Talk to your doctor about smoking cessation programs.

- If you're someone who drinks alcohol, drink in moderation.
- Remember your sunscreen. Use UV-AB-blocking sunscreen on your face and sunblock.
- Get vaccinated for human papillomavirus.
- Eat a well-balanced diet.
- Have regular **dental check-ups.** People between ages 20 and 40 should have an oral cancer screening every three years and annual exams after age 40.

Can I spot potential oral cancer?

Detecting oral cancer early can reduce the chance the cancer will grow or spread. You can detect oral cancer early by doing a monthly self-examination. If you spot changes or something unusual, contact your dentist immediately. Here's how to examine your mouth, throat and neck for signs of oral cancer:

- Feel your lips, the front of your gums and the roof of your mouth.
- Feel your neck and under your lower jaw for lumps or enlarged lymph nodes.
- Use a bright light and a mirror to look inside your mouth.
- Tilt your head back and look at the roof of your mouth.
- Pull your cheeks out to view the inside of your mouth, the lining of your cheeks and your back gums.
- Pull your tongue out and look at the top, bottom and sides. Gently push your tongue back so you can see the floor of your mouth.

- See for any kind of distinguish white, red or pigmented patch.
- Reduced mouth opening causing by hardening of cheek muscles.

What can I expect if I have oral cancer?

Oral cancer includes cancer in your mouth. Like most forms of cancer, early diagnosis and treatment improve the chance that oral cancer will spread. Approximately 1/3 of people treated for oral cancer develop new a cancer. If you've been treated for oral cancer, talk to your healthcare provider about follow-up examinations.

> **Make Dental Health Your Priority**

Periodontology

What does a periodontist do?

Periodontics is the specialty of dentistry which encompasses the prevention, diagnosis, and treatment of diseases of the supporting and surrounding tissues of the teeth or their substitutes and the replacement of lost teeth and supporting structures by regeneration, tissue engineering, and implantation of natural and/or synthetic devices and materials.

Problems Treated

- Bleeding gums
- Bad breath
- Pain on chewing
- Abscess
- Loosening of teeth
- Inflamed gums
- Receding gums

Procedures Performed

- Scaling and root planing
- Regenerative surgeries (bone and tissue grafts)
- Gingivectomy
- Crown lengthening
- Smile designing
- Dental implants
- Laser procedures

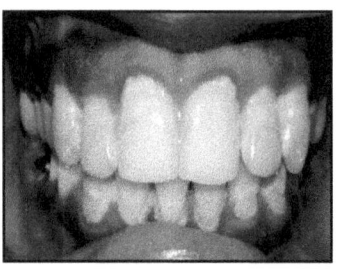

Gingivitis

Gingivitis is a common and mild form of gum disease (periodontal disease) that causes irritation, redness, and swelling (inflammation) of your gingiva, the part of your gum around the base of your teeth. It's important to take gingivitis seriously and treat it promptly. Gingivitis can lead to much more serious gum disease called periodontitis and tooth loss.

Healthy gums are firm and pale pink and fitted tightly around the teeth. Signs and symptoms of gingivitis include:

- Swollen or puffy gums
- Dusky red or dark red gums
- Gums that bleed easily when you brush or floss
- Bad breath
- Receding gums
- Tender gums

When to see a dentist

If you notice any signs and symptoms of gingivitis, schedule an appointment with your dentist. The sooner you seek care, the better your chances of reversing damage from gingivitis and preventing its progression to periodontitis.

Causes

The most common cause of gingivitis is poor oral hygiene which encourages plaque to form on teeth, causing inflammation of the surrounding gum tissues. Here's how plaque can lead to gingivitis:

- **Plaque forms on your teeth.** Plaque is an invisible, sticky film composed mainly of bacteria that forms on your teeth when starches and sugars in food interact with bacteria normally found in your mouth. Plaque requires daily removal because it re-forms quickly.
- **Plaque turns into tartar.** Plaque that stays on your teeth can harden under your gumline into tartar (calculus), which collects bacteria. Tartar makes plaque more difficult to remove, creates a protective shield for bacteria, and causes irritation along the gumline. You need professional dental cleaning to remove tartar.
- **Gingiva becomes inflamed (gingivitis).** The longer that plaque and tartar remain on your teeth, the more they irritate the gingiva, the part of your gum around the base of your teeth, causing inflammation. In time, your gums become swollen and bleed easily. Tooth decay (dental caries) also may result. If not treated, gingivitis can advance to periodontitis and eventual tooth loss.

Complications

Untreated gingivitis can progress to gum disease that spreads to underlying tissue and bone (periodontitis), a much more serious condition that can lead to tooth loss.

Chronic gingiva inflammation has been thought to be associated with some systemic diseases such as respiratory disease, diabetes, coronary artery disease, stroke and rheumatoid arthritis. Some research suggests that the bacteria responsible for periodontitis can enter your bloodstream through gum tissue, possibly affecting your heart, lungs and other parts of your body. But more studies are needed to confirm a link.

Trench mouth, also known as necrotizing ulcerative gingivitis (NUG), is a severe form of gingivitis that causes painful, infected, bleeding gums and ulcerations. Trench mouth is rare today in developed nations, though it's common in developing countries that have poor nutrition and poor living conditions.

The most common cause of gingivitis is poor oral hygiene. Good oral health habits, such as brushing at least twice a day, flossing daily and getting regular dental checkups, can help prevent and reverse gingivitis.

Treatment

GINGIVECTOMY/ GINGIVOPLASTY, which is the removal/ excision of the enlarged gingiva and reshaping to establish proper gingival shape (contours).

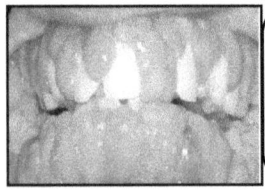

Drug Influenced Gingival Enlargement

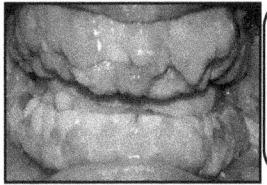

Gingival Enlargement Associated With Leukaemia

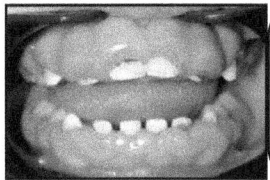

Hereditary Gingival Fibromatosis

Dental Plaque

What is dental plaque?

Dental plaque is a sticky film of bacteria that constantly forms on your teeth. It's normal to produce plaque. But if you don't remove plaque with routine dental cleanings and daily brushing and flossing, it can cause cavities, gum disease and other oral health issues.

What is tooth plaque made of?

Plaque contains bacteria, leftover food particles and saliva. When you eat, the bacteria in your mouth feed on food debris (like sugars and carbohydrates). This breaks the food down into a sticky, acidic film — what we know as dental plaque.

What does plaque look like on your teeth?

Technically, plaque is colourless. But sometimes it can cause tooth discoloration because food particles stick to the plaque.

Dental plaque makes your teeth look (and feel) "fuzzy." If you run your tongue over your teeth and it feels like they're wearing tiny sweaters, that's plaque.

What are the symptoms of dental plaque?

Common dental plaque symptoms include:

- A fuzzy feeling on your teeth.
- Bad breath (halitosis) that doesn't go away.
- Red, swollen gums that bleed after brushing.

How can I reduce dental plaque?

To reduce plaque, visit your dentist regularly and practice good oral hygiene.

Here's how to remove plaque from teeth:

- **Floss daily**. Floss once a day with dental floss to get rid of food and plaque stuck between teeth. Studies show that flossing before brushing teeth removes more plaque.
- **Brush twice a day**. Brush your teeth for two minutes with a soft-bristled toothbrush and fluoride toothpaste. Brush at least twice a day and preferably after every meal.
- **Chew sugarless gum**. If you can't brush soon after eating or drinking, chew sugar-free gum. Choose a kind that has the American Dental Association (ADA) Seal of Acceptance.
- **Choose healthy foods**. Cut back on sugary, starchy foods and drinks. Instead, choose nutritious foods and snacks such as plain yogurt, cheese, raw vegetables or fruit.

- **See your dentist**. Get dental checkups and cleanings at least twice a year.
- **Use mouthwash**. Rinse daily with an over-the-counter (OTC) or prescription antiseptic mouthwash.

What happens if plaque is not removed?

If you don't remove plaque through regular dental cleanings and daily brushing and flossing, it can cause serious dental conditions like cavities or gum disease. Proper oral hygiene and maintenance can help you prevent these issues.

Tartar (Dental Calculus)

What is tartar?

Tartar is hardened dental plaque that can form on your teeth, both above and below your gum line. Everybody gets plaque. But unless you remove it with proper oral hygiene, plaque can harden into tartar.

Unlike plaque, you can't remove tartar with brushing and flossing. A dentist or dental hygienist must remove it during a professional dental cleaning.

Another name for tartar is dental calculus.

What is tartar made of?

Tartar mostly contains dead bacteria that have mineralized, mixed with a small amount of mineralized proteins from your saliva (spit).

What are the symptoms of tartar on teeth?

If you start to develop tartar on your teeth, you might notice:

- Yellow, brown or black stains on your teeth.
- Bad breath (halitosis).
- Gingivitis (red, swollen or bleeding gums).
- A hard, crust-like coating on your teeth.

Does tartar smell bad?

Yes, tartar usually has an unpleasant odour. It can also cause small pockets to form in the areas between your teeth and gums. Bacteria and food debris can get trapped there, resulting in bad breath or a bad taste in your mouth.

What causes mouth tartar?

When you don't routinely remove plaque from your teeth, it can turn into tartar. So, tartar is usually a result of poor oral hygiene.

How do you treat tartar?

The only way to effectively treat tartar is to see a dentist or hygienist. They'll remove the tartar safely using a combination of special instruments.

It might be tempting to remove tartar from your teeth without a dentist, but this can actually damage your teeth and make you more susceptible to cavities and other issues.

Depending on the amount of tartar buildup you have, your dentist may recommend:

- Dental cleaning.
- Gum disease treatments.

Dental cleaning

Routine dental cleanings are the best way to keep your mouth and teeth healthy. During a cleaning, a dental hygienist removes plaque and tartar from your teeth using special instruments. They'll also thoroughly floss between your teeth and polish your teeth surfaces using a rubber cup and gritty toothpaste.

Many people can keep tartar at bay with cleanings every six months. But if you're prone to cavities, gum disease or other issues, you might need cleanings more often. Ask your dentist what cleaning schedule is right for you.

Gum disease treatments

If tartar has already caused some bone loss around your teeth, your dentist may recommend gum disease treatment. These procedures remove tartar that's trapped beneath your gum line, where brushing and flossing can't reach.

Common gum disease treatments include:

- Scaling and root planing.
- Osseous surgery (pocket reduction surgery).
- Laser periodontal therapy (using laser energy to kill bacteria under your gums).

How can I prevent tartar buildup?

To avoid issues like cavities and gum disease, it's best to stop tartar from forming in the first place. To help prevent tartar buildup on your teeth:

- **Brush your teeth two to three times every day.** Use a soft-bristled toothbrush and fluoride toothpaste.

(When you buy oral health products, make sure they have the American Dental Association, or ADA, Seal of Acceptance. This means they've passed rigorous tests for safety and effectiveness.)

- **Floss between your teeth once every day.** You can use traditional dental floss or tiny brushes that go in between your teeth. Ask your dentist or hygienist for specific product recommendations.
- **Swish with an alcohol-free, antibacterial mouthwash twice a day.** This helps kill oral bacteria that cause plaque and tartar buildup.
- **Avoid smoking and other tobacco products.** Research shows that people who smoke or chew tobacco have a much higher risk of developing tartar.
- **Visit your dentist regularly for exams and cleanings.** Brushing and flossing at home is essential for healthy teeth and gums. But you still need professional dental exams and cleanings. Many people do well with preventive visits twice a year. Others might need more frequent appointments. Ask your dentist what type of schedule is best for you.

What happens if I don't remove tartar?

If you leave tartar on your teeth, it can:

- Erode your enamel.
- Cause cavities.
- Make your gums swell and bleed.
- Lead to bad breath.
- Make your teeth look stained.

How often should I see my dentist for tartar removal?

It depends on your unique oral health needs. Some people build up plaque and tartar faster than others. Most people need cleanings every six months. But you might need them more often if you're prone to issues like tooth decay and gum disease. Ask your dentist what type of maintenance schedule is right for you.

Plaque vs. tartar: What's the difference?

Dental plaque is a yellowish, sticky film. It develops when bacteria in your mouth feed on sugars in the foods you eat. Plaque feels "fuzzy" on your teeth, but you can remove it with brushing and flossing.

Tartar is hardened plaque. It might be yellowish at first, but it can turn darker over time. Tartar feels like a hard shell on your teeth. Unlike plaque, you can't remove tartar with brushing and flossing.

Tooth Discoloration -

What is tooth discoloration?

Tooth discoloration refers to the staining or darkening of your teeth. You can develop discoloured teeth for a number of reasons. Some causes are unavoidable — like aging, trauma or disease. Other causes are preventable — like smoking and poor oral hygiene.

> Teeth can't fight cavities on their own so take care of it.

Types of tooth discoloration

There are two main types of tooth discoloration:

- **Extrinsic discoloration**: This type of discoloration affects the outer surface of your teeth (enamel). Exposure to certain environmental factors — like some foods and beverages — causes extrinsically discolored teeth.
- **Intrinsic discoloration**: This type of discoloration starts inside your tooth and affects your dentin (the layer underneath your enamel). Causes include dental trauma and certain medications.

What are the most common causes of discoloured teeth?

Several things can cause discoloured teeth. Some causes are avoidable. Others are unavoidable. Avoidable tooth discoloration causes include:

- **Dark-coloured foods and beverages**. Things like coffee, tea, cola drinks, red wine and soy sauce can stain your teeth over time.
- **Smoking and other tobacco use**. Research indicates that tooth discoloration is more common among people who smoke compared to people who don't.
- **Poor oral hygiene**. Stains cling to dental plaque. If you don't remove plaque with regular brushing and flossing, you're more likely to develop discoloured teeth.
- **Excessive fluoride**. In appropriate quantities, fluoride is an excellent way to protect your teeth from cavities. However, people who consume high levels of fluoride during childhood may develop fluorosis — a

condition that results in white spots on your tooth enamel.

Unavoidable tooth discoloration causes include:

- **Genetics**. Natural tooth colour, brightness and translucency vary from person to person.
- **Dental trauma**. Falls, car crashes and sports-related injuries can cause trauma that results in tooth discoloration.
- **Aging**. As you grow older, your tooth enamel wears thinner. This exposes more of the underlying dentin, which has a yellowish hue. As a result, your teeth may appear slightly more discoloured as you age.
- **Dental treatments**. Some dental materials — like silver amalgam used in metal fillings — can make your teeth appear greyish in colour. Root canal therapy can also cause tooth discoloration in some instances.
- **Certain diseases**. Some health conditions cause teeth discoloration, including liver disease, celiac disease, calcium deficiency, eating disorders and metabolic diseases.
- **Certain medications**. Some medications, like certain antihistamines and drugs for high blood pressure, can result in teeth discoloration. In addition, adults who took tetracycline or doxycycline (both antibiotics) during childhood may have tooth discoloration.
- **Cancer treatments**. Chemotherapy or head and neck radiation therapy can cause tooth discoloration.

Different colour meanings

Sometimes the colour of tooth stains can pinpoint the culprit:

- **Yellow** stains are usually due to eating and drinking dark-coloured foods or beverages. It may also mean that you need to improve your oral hygiene.
- **Brown** teeth discoloration is a result of smoking or using chewing tobacco. If you have brown stains and pitting (small holes) in your teeth, it probably means you have untreated tooth decay.
- **Purple** teeth stains usually affect people who consume a lot of red wine.
- **Gray** tooth discoloration may mean that the nerve inside your tooth has died. Dental trauma can cause this.
- **White** flecks on your teeth may indicate dental fluorosis. This means you consumed high levels of fluoride during childhood, when your teeth were developing.
- **Black** spots on your teeth typically indicate areas of severe decay.

How do dentists treat discoloured teeth?

Dentists use different tooth discoloration treatments depending on the underlying cause and whether the stains affect the outer or inner layers of your teeth.

Teeth whitening

Dentists may offer in-office or at-home professional teeth whitening treatments. These methods use hydrogen peroxide or carbamide peroxide to break up stains and lift them from your teeth. Professional whitening works best on surface (extrinsic) stains. But some whitening products can remove deep dental (intrinsic) stains, too.

In-office bleaching takes about one hour to complete. Most take-home whitening treatments require 30- to 60-minute daily treatments for up to six weeks. There are pros and cons to each. Ask your dentist which option is right for you.

Dental bonding

If you have deep tooth discoloration that doesn't improve with whitening, your dentist may recommend dental bonding. This procedure involves applying tooth-coloured composite resin to conceal discoloured teeth.

Bonding is much more affordable compared to other options (like porcelain veneers), but you'll probably need touch-ups every five to seven years. Dental bonding might not be the best option if you have several discoloured teeth.

Porcelain veneers

If you have widespread tooth discoloration that doesn't improve with whitening, you may want to consider porcelain veneers. These tooth-coloured ceramic shells are thin, yet strong. A dentist permanently bonds (glues) them to the front surfaces of your teeth to camouflage discoloration or other cosmetic flaws like chipping or misshapen teeth.

A dentist has to replace porcelain veneers every five to 15 years. Veneers aren't reversible.

Dental crowns

Sometimes tooth discoloration is a symptom of cavities. If you have weakened or decayed teeth in addition to discoloration, your dentist may recommend dental crowns.

A crown is a tooth-shaped cap that fits over your tooth, protecting it from further damage. Dental crowns help improve the health and function of your teeth as well as their appearance.

How can I fix discoloured teeth at home?

You can find over-the-counter (OTC) teeth whitening treatments in any oral health aisle. These products include rinses, pastes, strips and do-it-yourself bleaching trays.

While some over-the-counter products are safe and effective, others can damage your enamel and make your teeth more vulnerable to cavities and erosion. That's why it's important to talk to your dentist before making a purchase.

In general, ingredients to avoid include:

- Baking soda (sodium bicarbonate).
- Activated charcoal.
- Citric acid.

When shopping for teeth whitening products, look for the ADA Seal of Acceptance. This means that experts have tested the safety and effectiveness of these products and deemed them safe for use.

Can I prevent tooth discoloration?

While you can't prevent deep dental stains due to trauma, medications or health conditions, there are things you can do to reduce your risk of everyday surface discoloration:

- Brush your teeth two to three times a day using a soft-bristled brush and ADA-approved fluoride toothpaste.
- Floss between your teeth once a day.
- Limit foods and drinks that stain teeth, like tea, coffee, cola and red wine.
- Drink lots of water and rinse your mouth after drinking beverages that could cause tooth discoloration.
- Quit smoking and visit your dentist for routine examinations.

Orthodontics

ORTHODONTIST: A dentist for your crooked teeth

The term "orthodontics" can be broken down into two Greek words - "orthos" meaning straight or correct and "dontics" meaning teeth.

What Does An Orthodontist Do?

Orthodontics, therefore describes the practice of straightening misaligned teeth or malocclusions. Dentists who specialize in orthodontics can help manage abnormal positioning of the teeth, jaws, and face.

> **Father of modern Orthodontics- Edward Hartley Angle.**

Benefits of Orthodontics

Orthodontics has additional benefits over improving cosmetic appearance. The benefits of opting for straightening the teeth include:

- Improvement of self-esteem
- Improved function of teeth including better chewing and clearer pronunciation and speech
- Reduced risk of dental caries occurring due to the collection of food particles between the teeth
- Reduced risk of gum injury and trauma due to overbites and malocclusions

Aims of orthodontic treatment

- Providing cosmetic correction and improving the appearance.
- Providing a healthy functional bite.
- Preventing diseases of the teeth.

Problems Treated-

Some of the dental malocclusions that may be corrected by orthodontics include:

- Crowded teeth - Crowding of teeth or poor alignment of teeth that may be too large for the mouth. This leads to a poor bite as well as an unsightly appearance. The most common teeth to crowd are the upper canine teeth.
- An open bite - This occurs when the lower end of the upper front teeth does not touch the upper end of the lower front teeth. This leads to insufficient chewing.
- Deep overbite - This describes when the top and bottom front teeth are not aligned and the bottom teeth tend to touch the roof of the mouth, sometimes damaging the gums and the palate. This may lead to gum damage, gum diseases, tooth loss, and tooth wear.
- Crossbite - This occurs when the teeth end does not meet. It leads to poor appearance, insufficient chewing, and easily erodible teeth.
- Increased overjet - This describes when the upper teeth protrude and may result from thumb or finger sucking. This may also be due to uneven jaw bone growth.

- Reverse overjet - The lower jaw protrudes beyond the upper jaw. Aside from poor cosmetic appearance, it can lead to worn teeth.
- Spacing - Unnatural spacing between teeth may result from poorly developed, smaller or missing teeth.

Procedure Performed-

Teeth can be straightened in adults, adolescents, or children, using braces that may be fixed or removable. These may be

Removable Appliances

These are the devices that can be inserted into and removed from the oral cavity by the patient's will.

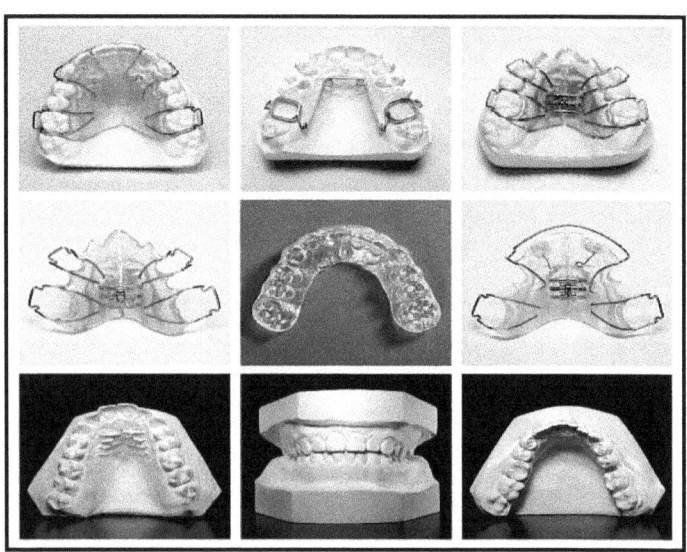

Fixed Appliances

These are the devices that are attached to the teeth, cannot be removed by the patient, and can cause tooth movement.

Fixed appliance treatment is the most precise way to control tooth movement to achieve the perfect smile. There are three main components to such appliances including the brackets (which are attached to the teeth), arch wires (the wires placed into the brackets) and auxiliaries such as elastics.

metal or ceramic brackets glued to the front teeth and stainless-steel bands cemented around the back teeth. These components are connected by a horseshoe-shaped arch wires.

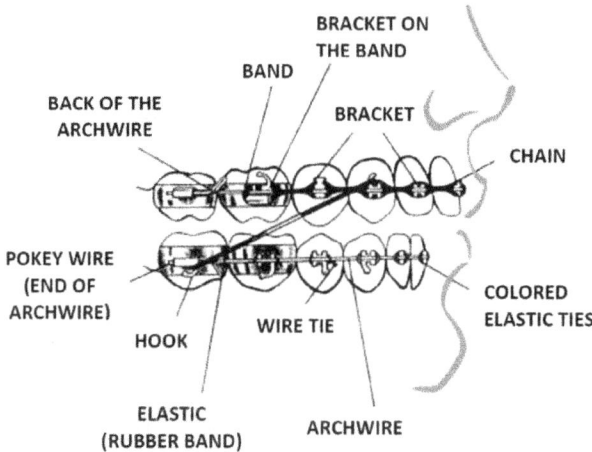

Orthodontic Food List

There are certain dietary habits that are known to cause breakage of orthodontic appliances as well as increase the risk of dental disease. Our aim is to achieve the treatment goals with as few disturbances due to appliance breakage as possible and to minimize the side effects of poor diet choices. Remember, teeth move best in a healthy environment and in individuals with excellent overall health. Be sure you have a well-balanced diet.

Potential harm to your teeth and gums

Foods and drinks which your dentist has suggested may cause dental caries (cavities) should be restricted while wearing braces. Sticky foods are to be avoided because of the increased risk of dental decay and appliance breakage. These foods stick to braces and remain on your teeth for long periods of time. If foods or drinks high in sugar content are to be consumed, we advise having them with regular meals or at one given time of day. Please make sure that careful brushing and rinsing take place immediately afterwards. Between meal snacks should be confined to foods without refined sugar and should be followed by vigorous rinsing if a toothbrush is not available.

Please keep fingers and pencils away from your brackets. Avoid "picking" at your braces to avoid harm to the appliances.

> **The Orthodontic Bracket Was Invented by Edward Angle In 1915**

Potential harm to your braces

Braces are attached to your teeth with an adhesive which normally will withstand the forces of eating. However, braces can be dislodged and wires bent or broken while eating certain foods. Hard foods, such as nuts, hard candy, corn chips and even crisp taco shells, can harm your braces and should be avoided. Chewing ice cubes, pencils and fingernails can also be very destructive to your appliances. Some foods, such as whole apples, raw carrots or celery, are healthy snacks, but must be cut up to avoid damaging your braces.

Chewy foods, such as gum, caramels, and even thick bread crusts, can bend and distort wires causing treatment delays and extra visits for repairs. Popcorn can cause harm in multiple ways. The husks from the popcorn can become lodged beneath the braces and cause irritation to the gum tissue. Un-popped kernels can shear or break off brackets as well as bend or dislodge wires.

Oral and Maxillofacial Surgery

What Does An Oral Surgeon Do?

An oral surgeon performs any surgical procedure on your teeth, gums, jaws or other oral structures. This includes extractions, implants, gum grafts and jaw surgeries.

Problem Treated-

- Extensive tooth decay.
- badly broken teeth.
- Gum disease.
- Impacted teeth.
- Missing teeth.
- Temporomandibular joint disorders (TMD).
- Bone loss in your jaw.
- Sleep apnea.
- Oral cancer., etc.

Procedure Performed-

Extractions.

Dental bone graft.

Dental implants.

Corrective jaw surgery.

Cleft lip and palate repair.

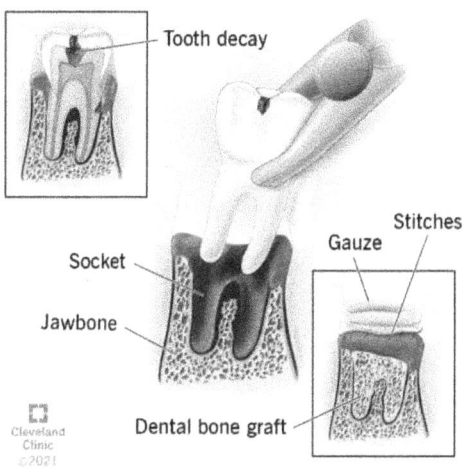

Tooth Extraction

Tooth Extraction

A tooth extraction may be necessary for many reasons, including severe damage or decay. One of the most common dental procedures, tooth extraction can eliminate bacteria and improve your overall oral health.

What is a tooth extraction?

A tooth extraction is a dental procedure during which your tooth is completely removed from its socket.

When is tooth extraction recommended?

Healthcare providers prefer to save natural teeth whenever possible. But sometimes, other restorative methods — such as dental fillings or dental crowns — aren't enough. If your tooth has been badly damaged past the point of repair, then removal may be necessary. Your dentist may recommend tooth extraction if you have:

- Severe tooth decay (cavities).
- A fractured tooth.
- An impacted tooth.
- Crowded teeth.
- Severe gum disease.
- Tooth luxation or other dental injuries.

Who performs tooth extraction?

Dentists and some dental specialists — such as oral surgeons and periodontists — can perform tooth extractions. While general dentists perform plenty of extractions, more complex cases are usually referred out to oral surgeons or periodontists.

What happens before a tooth extraction?

Your dentist will assess your affected tooth and surrounding gums. Your dentist will also take dental X-rays to check bone levels and determine the extent of damage. Be sure to tell your dentist about any medications, vitamins, or supplements you're taking.

What happens during a tooth extraction?

First, local anesthesia is given to numb your affected tooth and surrounding gum tissue. Using specialized dental instruments, your dentist will gently loosen your tooth and carefully lift it from its socket. Sometimes, your dentist might need to make incisions in your gums to access your tooth — especially if your tooth is badly decayed or has broken off at the gum line. Once your tooth is removed, the socket is cleaned and disinfected. In some cases, your dentist may also place a dental bone graft, which helps prevent bone loss in your jaw. Finally, stitches may be placed to help promote healing.

What happens after a tooth extraction?

When the procedure is complete, your dentist will place a piece of gauze over the extraction site and ask you to close it down with firm, steady pressure. This helps slow bleeding so a blood clot can form. (Clotting is a normal aspect of recovery. It promotes healing and reduces the risk of dry sockets.) You'll take the gauze out once the bleeding has slowed enough. You may continue to have light bleeding throughout the first 24 hours.

> **James Garretson (1825-1895) is the father of oral surgery.**

What are the advantages of pulling a tooth?

Tooth extraction offers several benefits. Most importantly, it reduces harmful bacteria that can damage your teeth and gums. Left untreated, a decayed or damaged tooth can wreak havoc on your smile, causing a domino effect of problems. Removing your affected tooth gives you the best chance for optimal oral health. Additionally, tooth extraction can help ease dental pain almost immediately — especially if your tooth was severely broken or infected.

What are the risks or complications of tooth extraction?

Like any surgical procedure, tooth extraction carries a small risk of complications. These may include:

- Post-surgical infection.
- Dry socket.
- Nerve injury.
- Perforation of maxillary sinus.
- Delayed healing.

What are the side effects of removing a tooth?

Normal side effects following tooth extraction include bleeding, swelling and discomfort. Your dentist will provide instructions on how to successfully manage your healing. How long does it take to recover from a tooth extraction?

It depends on the complexity of your case. However, most people feel back to normal in just a few days. While you'll be able to return to routine activities within 48 to 72 hours, it usually takes the jawbone several weeks to heal completely. Therefore, if you're planning on replacing the tooth with a dental implant, you'll probably need to wait a few months to allow for full recovery.

10 Things You Did Not Know About Wisdom Teeth!

1. Wisdom teeth are the third and final set of molars that most people get in their late teens or early twenties.
2. When wisdom teeth are misaligned, they may position themselves horizontally or be angled.
3. Poor alignment of wisdom teeth can crowd or damage adjacent teeth, the jaw bone or nerve.
4. Wisdom teeth also can be impacted many times within the soft tissue or jawbone or only partially erupt through gum.

5. Partial eruption allows an opening for bacteria to enter around the tooth and cause infection, which results in pain, swelling, jaw stiffness, difficulty in mouth opening.
6. Wisdom teeth do not always have to be removed. They are only extracted when they are impacted or causing other issues
7. Not everyone actually has wisdom teeth. Some people have them beneath the gums, some people have one or two and some people don't have any.
8. The greatest of all myths is Wisdom teeth removal causes vision disturbances. No removing upper teeth or for that matter any teeth effect a person's eyesight. The nerves which supply eyes and teeth are different hence, no interconnection.
9. Through dental x-rays or routine check-ups dentist can keep a tab on the wisdom teeth. Unfortunately, it is not possible to predict way that wisdom teeth will erupt.
10. Not always Wisdom tooth extraction is painful and complicated. Upper molars are easier to remove than lower molars it all depends on the tooth anatomy, curvature of the roots and location of the teeth either it is erupted or impacted. Effective local anaesthesia renders least amount of pain to the patients. The local anaesthesia desensitizes a patient to pain during an extraction so that there is not much discomfort while removal of teeth. Note that there may be some amount of pain after the procedure.

Tooth extraction aftercare

After your extraction, your dentist will give you a detailed list of post-surgical instructions. Here are some general guidelines for a speedy recovery:

- **Keep the extraction site clean.** Gently rinse the area with an antimicrobial mouthwash two to three times a day. Avoid brushing directly over your extraction site until your dentist tells you it's safe to do so. Brush and floss all other areas normally.
- **Take all medications as directed.** Your dentist may prescribe antibiotics and pain relievers. It's important to take all of these medications exactly as directed. You can also take over-the-counter pain relievers, such as acetaminophen and ibuprofen.
- **Avoid strenuous activity for at least two days.** An elevated heart rate can cause increased post-operative bleeding and discomfort. Skip the gym for the first 48 to 72 hours. Ask your dentist when it's safe to resume normal routines.

What can I eat after a tooth extraction?

Avoid hard and crunchy foods for the first few days. Stock your fridge and pantry with soft foods like rice, pasta, eggs, yogurt and applesauce. You'll also want to avoid drinking through straws, as this can dislodge blood clots and cause dry sockets.

> **Take all of your medications as per the surgeon instruction.**

Pedodontics

Pedodontist: A Dentist for Children

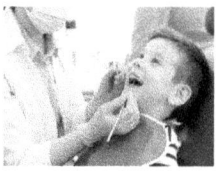

Paediatric dentists are professionals who have completed a specialized course of dentistry that caters to children who have special needs or otherwise need gentle care. The program consists of three years of further training after graduation from dental school. It includes hospital training, where they work with children who have more severe dental needs and emergencies, and training in numerous orthodontic teeth-straightening methods. Paediatric dentists work closely with paediatricians and general dentists, who refer select patients for this specialized dental treatment that requires this advanced training.

What Does a Paediatric Dentist Do?

Pedodontics is a dental specialty that deals with the care of children's teeth. It is also spelled as pedodontics. The pedodontics is concerned with prevention, which includes instruction in a proper diet, fluoride use, and oral hygiene practices. The pedodontist's routine practice focuses on caries (tooth decay), but it also includes influencing tooth alignment. To correct early abnormalities in tooth position, lengthy treatment may be required. Braces or other types of correctional devices may be used.

> Be the role model of the child by practicing healthy oral hygiene

Aim-

Paediatric dentists perform a variety of important functions related to a child's overall oral health and hygiene. They place a special emphasis on the proper maintenance and care of deciduous (baby) teeth, which are important in facilitating good chewing habits, proper speech production, and also holding space for permanent teeth.

Other important functions include:

Education – Paediatric dentists educate children using models, computer technology, and child-friendly terminology, emphasizing the importance of keeping teeth strong and healthy. They also counsel parents on disease prevention, trauma prevention, healthy eating habits, and other aspects of household hygiene.

Monitoring Growth – Paediatric dentists can anticipate dental issues and intervene quickly before they worsen by continuously tracking growth and development. Working toward earlier corrective treatment also helps to maintain the child's self-esteem and promotes a more positive self-image.

Prevention – Helping parents, as well as children, establish sound eating and oral care habits

Pedodontics Treatment

It is strongly advised in pedodontics treatment that all young children be examined by a paediatric dentist from an early age. The first step in treatment is the patient's first dental checkup. As a general rule, young children should see a dentist as soon as their first tooth appears, or by the time the child is one year old. These early visits inform parents of whether they're properly cleaning their child's teeth at home.

Following the initial visit, regular checkups every six months should be scheduled. Patients will have routine teeth cleaning and dental exams during these regular checkups. A fluoride treatment may also be administered by the dentist on a regularly to protect against tooth decay caused by sugars and bacteria.

In the course of pedodontics treatment, the dentist may need to perform several procedures, including the few procedures listed below:

1. **Fillings** – This entails removing any decayed or damaged tooth structure. After that, the hole is filled with metal, plastic, or other filling materials. The procedure keeps the decay from worsening and spreading further into the tooth.

2. **Extractions** – Tooth extractions are done when a tooth is severely damaged or infected, or when a child's teeth are overcrowded.

3. **Dental Crowns** – Dental crowns may also be required for young children to restore badly damaged teeth. The procedure begins with the removal of caries or cavities and the reduction of the size of the tooth to accommodate the crown.

4. **Root Canals** – Root canals are typically used to treat decayed or infected teeth, as well as injuries that result in tooth loss.

5. **Dental X-rays** – Dental X-rays are a standard part of a routine dental exam. Dentists can use X-rays to detect bone damage, tooth decay, impacted teeth, and dental injuries, among other potentially serious issues.

6. **Sealants** – Once children start getting their molars, dentists may recommend the use of sealants which

generally protect the surface of the teeth from wear as well as tear.

Pedodontics treatment may also include oral as well as maxillofacial surgery, orthodontics, periodontics, and prosthodontics in some cases. Orthodontics, for example, is most commonly performed during a child's adolescent years because this is the best time to ensure that the teeth and jawbones are properly aligned.

Robert Bunon- Father of Pediatric Dentistry

The First Teeth to Erupt Is the Lower Central Incisor.

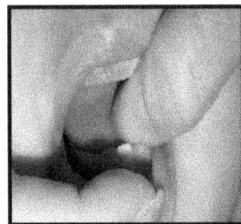

Most babies will develop teeth between 6 and 12 months.

Natal/ Neonatal Tooth

Very rarely an infant may be born with a tooth in their oral cavity usually in the lower jaw. These teeth are very small, not fully developed, and may be loose. This condition need not be considered an abnormality, as usually, the tooth is a part of the normal dentition.

NO TREATMENT USUALLY REQUIRED.

EXTRACTION -only if -

1. Tooth is loose enough that it may be aspirated

2. Tooth is causing hindrance in feeding.

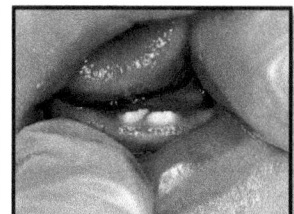

> **A Baby Tooth Won't Fall Out Unless There's an Adult Tooth to Replace It.**

Nursing Bottle Caries/ Early Childhood Caries

Usually occurs in children aged 0-3 years.

Cause – bottle feeding at night with sweetened milk/ liquid and not rising it afterward, leaving it like that overnight helps bacteria to cause caries.

Common sites –upper incisors and first molars Seen as circumferential lesions which progress at a rapid rate. The lower teeth remain mostly unaffected.

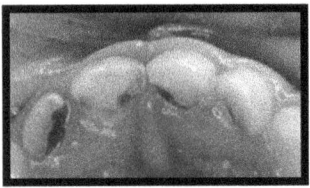 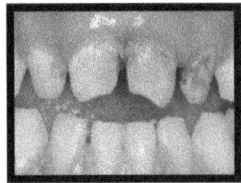

Visit The Dentist In Every 6 Months.

Ugly Duckling Stage

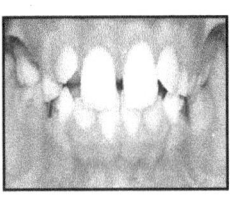 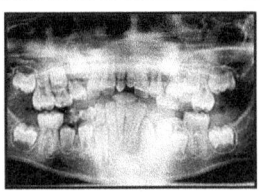

As the developing canine erupts, they displace the roots of the lateral incisor mesially.

This results in transmitting of the force onto the roots of the central incisors which also get displaced mesially.

A resultant distal divergence of the crowns of the two central incisors causes a midline spacing.

This situation has been described by Broadbent as the ugly-duckling stage.

Cleft Lip and Cleft Palate

What is cleft lip and palate?

CLEFT MEANS GAP. A cleft lip is a separation of the two sides of the lip. The separation often includes the bones of the upper jaw and/or upper gum. A cleft palate is an opening in the roof of the mouth. Cleft lip and palate is a condition, which occurs when the two sides of the lip or roof of the mouth (palate) do not completely fuse, as the unborn baby was developing. The lip and palate develop separately so a child can have a cleft lip, a cleft palate, or both. The size of the cleft lip may range from a small notch in the upper lip to an opening that extends into the base of the nostril. The cleft may be single-sided or may occur on both sides.

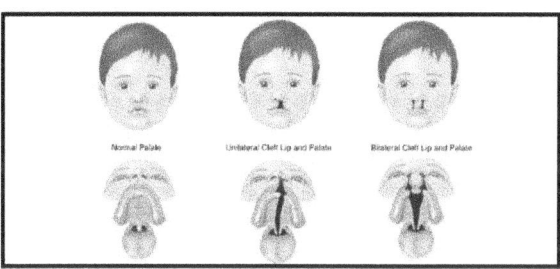

Having a baby born with a cleft can be upsetting, but cleft lip and cleft palate can be corrected. In most babies, a series of surgeries can restore normal function and achieve a more normal appearance with minimal scarring.

> **Eat a balanced diet to keep teeth healthy.**

How to make feeding easy for a child with a cleft palate?

1-Use a Squeeze soft bottle

2-Conventional nipple can be modified by making the hole big enough so that milk drips down drop by drop without much effort.

Feeding Position

- Mother should hold the baby in the lap at about 45°, keeping his head high so that milk/feed does not get into the lungs.
- Use small feeds each time
- Frequent Burping should be initiated following the feed
- The Use of a deep spoon can be useful

How does this help the child?

- The Child is unable to create negative pressure because of the defect in the palate and hence cannot suck the milk from the nipple.
- A Big hole in the nipple helps drip the milk effortlessly
- Drip the milk in the area of the intact palate, watch for milk getting down for the child to swallow. It should not get into the breathing tube or come out of the nose.

Treatments

Basically, surgery for cleft lips/palate is planned in many stages depending on the severity.

3 months-primary surgery

the purpose of surgery is to close the gap in the lip and also the front part of the palate

9 months to 1 year- Palate Repair (secondary surgery)

1-To close the back part of the palate down up to the soft palate.

2-Revision of lip and deepening of sulcus when the upper lip is not very mobile

3-To develop good speech both upper and lower lip should meet

6 years- 9 years final check-up

1-To check for irregularities of teeth.

2-To check the quality of speech development.

9 years -12 years

1- Have Speech improvement taken place or not.?

2-Does fluid escape from mouth to nose.?

18 years and above

Scar revision or rhinoplasty Rehabilitation of missing teeth

MILESTONES TO GOOD OUTCOME

Cleft children are not different from other kids.

- They can grow and live normally.

A Cleft Surgeon is your friend

- Do not forget to see him at regular intervals

- Do not see him only when you need surgery

Consult Speech Therapist

- He may guide you for speech and hearing problems

- Follow timings of treatment 6 months to 2 years are critical for speech.

Consult orthodontist

- 6 years and above orthodontic consultation is important

It is our responsibility to make the life of a cleft baby a blessing!

Conservative and Endodontic Dentistry

What does an endodontist do?

An endodontist is a dental specialist who focuses on complex tooth problems that primarily affect tooth pulp. Tooth "pulp" is what dental providers call the nerves, blood vessels and other tissues deep inside each tooth. When you look in the mirror, the part of your teeth you see is an outer layer called enamel.

Endodontists use advanced techniques to treat dental pulp and root issues. Your root is the part of your tooth that extends below your gums and holds your tooth in place. Endodontists focus on relieving tooth or mouth pain while saving your natural tooth whenever possible.

Common reasons to see an endodontist

Endodontists primarily treat damaged tooth pulp or root tissues arising from the following causes:

- **Tooth decay**: the breakdown of a tooth that results from poor teeth and gum care (oral hygiene). You may see an endodontist if an untreated cavity damages your tooth's root tissues. Tooth decay can cause inflammation (pulpitis) or even death (necrosis) and infection in the pulp tissue.

> Care for children should be done by observing their behavior management.

- **Tooth injuries**: Trauma affecting your tooth (such as from a hard fall).
- **Tooth abscess**: A buildup of pus that forms when bacteria get inside your tooth or gums.
- **Cracked tooth**: Damage to your tooth that allows an opening for bacteria to get inside.

Endodontics procedures

Endodontists are sometimes called root canal dentists. While general dentists and endodontists both perform root canal treatment, endodontists perform this procedure much more often. The additional training and higher treatment volume mean that endodontists are the experts in doing root canals.

Endodontists perform multiple procedures:

- **Root canal**: Removes damaged or infected tooth pulp and reseals the tooth to prevent reinfection.
- **Endodontic retreatment**: Removes and replaces materials from a previous root canal that didn't heal properly.
- **Endodontic surgery**: Specialized surgery, such as apicoectomy (removal of the end, or tip, of a tooth's root).
- **Emergency dental surgery**: This may involve repairing complex dental injuries or treating severe tooth infections.
- **Tooth extraction (removal) surgery**: Pulling a tooth because there's too much tissue damage for a provider to save it.

- **Dental implant surgery**: Surgical placement of a dental implant. A provider can use the implant to support prosthetics, such as bridges, and restore the look and function of your teeth after you have a tooth removed.

All endodontists are also dentists, which means they may perform the same procedures common in general dentistry, including cleaning, whitening, veneer, crown and others.

How does an endodontist test a tooth?

Endodontists have specialized training to diagnose many complex causes of tooth, mouth (oral) and facial pain. An endodontist may check your symptoms by performing one or more tests:

- **Dental X-rays**: Capture clear details of tooth structures.
- **Hot or cold swabs**: Test your tooth's sensitivity when it comes into contact with different temperatures.
- **Tapping on teeth**: This May provide clues to what tooth has inflammation and how far the inflammation has spread, especially if your teeth are sensitive to the tapping.

Avoid smoking and tobacco products.

Dental Caries/ Tooth Decay/ Cavity

Dental caries is the breakdown of the tooth structure due to the acids produced by the bacteria, that cause demineralization of the inorganic portion and degradation of the organic matter. It is multifactorial and is dependent on the type of diet, presence of bacterial microorganisms and maintenance of hygiene.

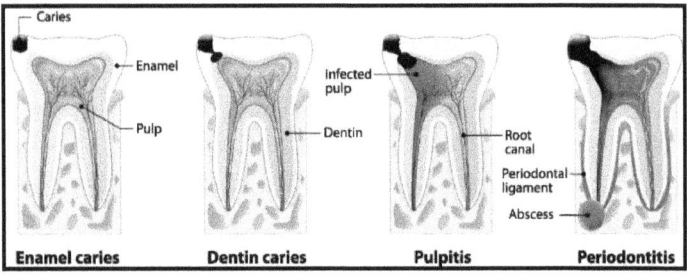

Eat a healthy balanced diet.

Restoration / Fillings

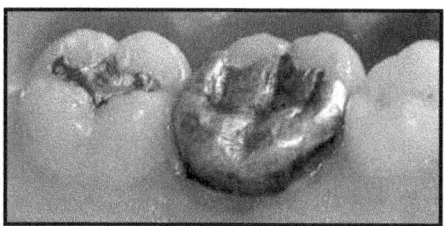

Amalgam Restorations

Advantages

1. High compressive strength
2. Wear resistance
3. Economic
4. Self-sealing abilities
5. Durable

Disadvantages –

1. Not an aesthetic option
2. Extensive cavity preparation
3. Non – insulating
4. Prone to tarnish & corrosion

> **Teeth start to form before we are born.**

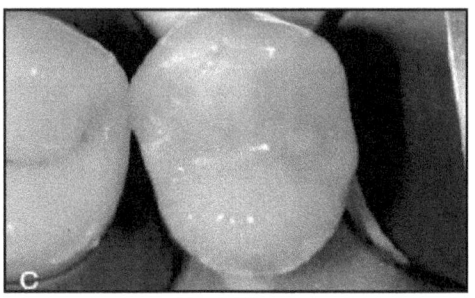

Composite Restoration

Advantages –

1. Aesthetics
2. Conservation of tooth structure
3. Good adhesion to tooth
4. Repairable
5. Durable

Disadvantages

1. Technique sensitive
2. Expensive

> Tooth decay is the second most common disease after cold.

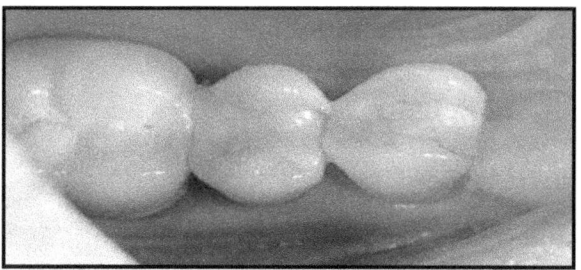

Glass Ionomer Cement Restoration

Advantages –

1. Adhesion to tooth
2. Anti-cariogenic effect
3. Biocompatibility
4. Good aesthetics
5. Not technique sensitive
6. Semi-durable

Disadvantages –

1. Low fracture and wear resistance

> **Make it a routine for brushing twice daily.**

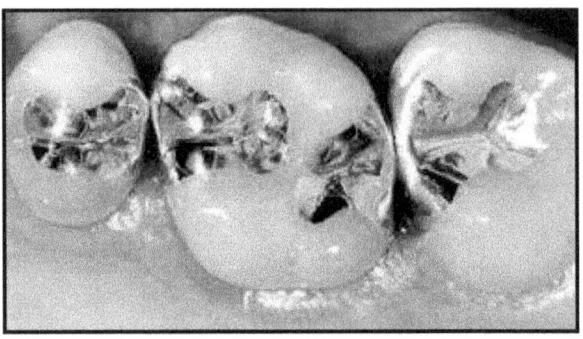

Gold Restoration

Advantages –

1. Durable
2. Tarnish & corrosion resistant
3. Insoluble to oral fluids
4. No plaque accumulation

Disadvantages-

1. Not very aesthetic
2. Time-consuming
3. Very Expensive

> Keep tongue clean.

Root Canal Therapy (RCT)

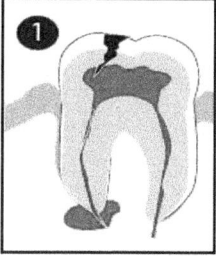

Infected pulp tissue

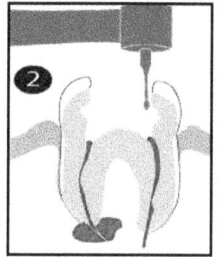

Access opening (removal of the infected tissue)

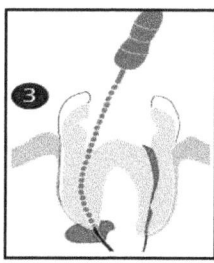

Cleaning and shaping of canals.

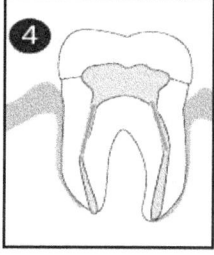

Obturation

(filling of canals with suitable material and restoration of crown structure)

Procedures maybe performed at separate appointments **(Multiple visit or Conventional Endodontics)** or at a single appointment **(Single visit endodontics)**.

RCT should be done when **DIAGNOSTIC RADIOGRAPH** shows radiolucency extending to the pulp

Radiograph showing normal tooth structure with no caries

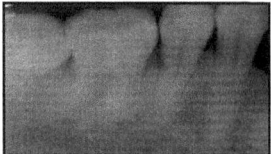

Radiograph showing caries (radiolucency) extending to the pulp chamber. Hence, RCT of the tooth is required

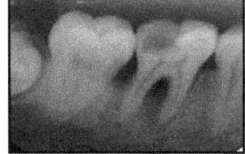

When can single-visit RCT be performed?

- RCT of an uncomplicated vital tooth
- Fractured anterior or bicuspid which is aesthetically important
- Accidental mechanical pulp exposure
- Medically compromised patients requiring prophylactic antibiotics
- Physically challenged individuals

Smile as it suits you.

When single visit RCT cannot be performed?

- Presence of pain on percussion
- Pus discharge is present
- Limited access to the tooth
- Calcified and curved canals are present
- Patients with TMJ disorder

Dental Bleaching

Bleaching is the lightening of the discolorations of teeth through the application of chemical agents. It can be done in the dental office as well as at home.

When to go for bleaching?

1. Slight tobacco/ tea/coffee stains are present
2. Mild brownish stains due to fluorosis/ tetracycline

When to avoid bleaching?

1. If teeth appear naturally yellow due to thin enamel
2. If teeth are sensitive to cold fluid/ food
3. Presence of severe fluorosis with enamel pitting

Broken teeth can be saved.

Things to keep in mind about bleaching

1. Hypersensitivity may develop after bleaching, especially if the enamel is thin.

2. Do not expect heavy stains to disappear. Bleaching is best suited for mild stains only. Very heavy stains may become slightly lighter.

3. Your dentist may advise a combination of bleaching and composite restoration/ veneers to provide better aesthetic results.

Tip: brush in small circles.

Draw tiny "O" on your teeth

Prosthodontics

Prosthodontics is the dental specialty about the diagnosis, treatment planning, rehabilitation and maintenance of the oral function, comfort, appearance and health of patients with clinical conditions associated with missing or deficient teeth and/ or maxillofacial tissues using biocompatible substitutes.

Problems Treated

- Missing tooth
- Multiple missing teeth
- Palatal defects
- Enucleated eye
- Loss of external structure of nose/ ear

Procedures Performed

- Crown
- Complete dentures
- Removable partial dentures
- Fixed partial dentures
- Complete oral rehabilitation
- Implant-supported prosthesis
- Night guard for TMJ disorder and sleep apnea
- Cranio-Facial Prosthesis (eye)
- Other prosthesis (Finger

> **Rinse your mouth with water after every meal.**

Missing Tooth and Its Effects

The most major and obvious effect of tooth loss is loss in masticatory abilities, but besides that various other changes are observed after tooth loss.

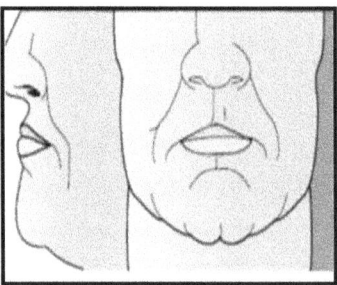

Aesthetic changes – decrease in facial height and deepening of vertical lines

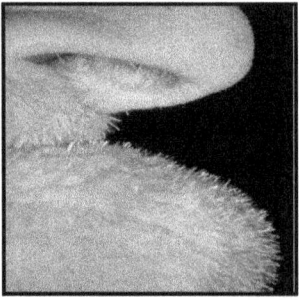

Decrease in vertical height leading to tilting of chin

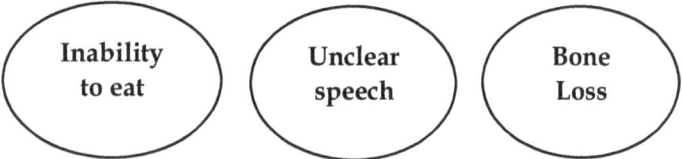

Causes of Tooth Loss / Tooth Replacement Options

- Dental caries
- Periodontal disease
- Tooth fracture/accidents/trauma

Replacement Options for Complete Tooth Loss

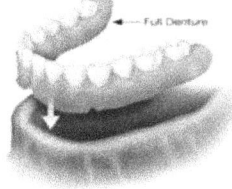 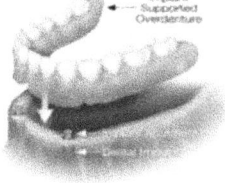

Complete / Full Denture   Overdenture

Denture tip: Clean your dentures every day.

Replacement Options for Partial/ Single Tooth Loss

Removable Partial Denture

Missing teeth are replaced using acrylic teeth and denture base, similar to complete dentures. Clasps (metal hooks) may be given for added retention. These are removable prosthesis

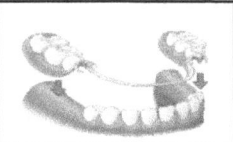

Fixed Partial Denture

One or more than one tooth can be replaced and it is a fixed prosthetic option. Teeth adjacent to the missing teeth are used as support (abutments) to support the prosthesis.

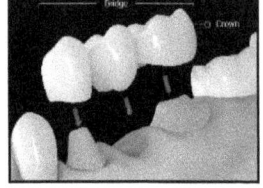

It can be given only when the supporting teeth (abutments) are firm, have proper bony support and the ability to withstand additional forces. These require proper hygiene maintenance as the area is more prone to food lodgement

> Dental crown functions as a permanent restoration of tooth's shape, size and strength.

Tooth Replacement by Dental Implants

A dental implant is a fixture which is inserted into the alveolar bone and it acts as a replacement of the root of the tooth. This portion is submerged within the bone and is not visible after completion of the surgery. Over this fixture (dental implant) a component (abutment) is placed which acts as a platform for the placement of a crown (that replaces the crown of the tooth).

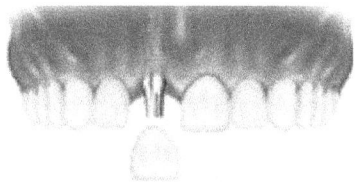

Single tooth replacement with an implant

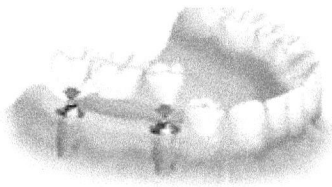

Multiple tooth replacement with an implant.

Dental Crown / Cap

A dental crown/cap is a form of restoration that covers or encircles the entire crown portion of the tooth made of dental materials such as metal, ceramic, or porcelain.

Is a dental crown necessary after RCT?

Yes, a dental crown is necessary after RCT, as after RCT the tooth loses its resilience and becomes brittle and thus, more prone to fracture. A crown helps protect the tooth and reinforces strength and therefore should be placed as soon as possible after the RCT.

What is done for crown placement?

The dentist will first reduce the natural tooth present and make the tooth smaller, so that the crown can be placed easily. This is done so that when the crown is placed it resembles the natural tooth as closely as possible and there is no bulkiness which would otherwise lead to discomfort.

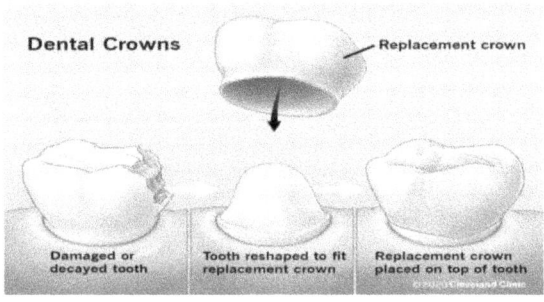

What are some other situations where you might be advised a crown?

A canal is a definite indication of the crown. Apart from this, a dentist may advise crowns for aesthetic purposes where the patient desires an improvement in the shape/ proclination or color of his /their teeth. It may also be advised when a tooth has lost its strength due to pathological reasons

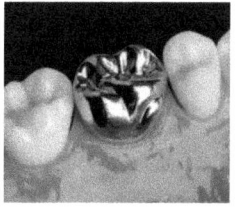

Full coverage crowns made of metal.

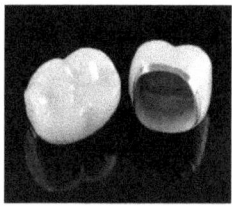

Crowns made of porcelain fused to metal i.e. a base of metal over which porcelain is fired

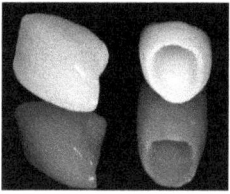

All ceramic crowns – manufactured using CAD-CAM machine

Each tooth has a job to do.

Oral Pathology

What Oral Pathology means?

Oral pathology is the specialty of dentistry and discipline of pathology that deals with the nature, identification, and management of diseases affecting the oral and maxillofacial regions.

What Oral Pathologist do?

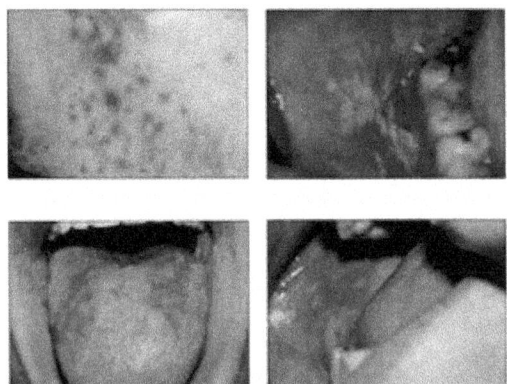

The specialty **oral and maxillofacial pathology** is concerned with diagnosis and study of the causes and effects of diseases affecting the oral and maxillofacial region. It is sometimes considered to be a specialty of dentistry and pathology. Sometimes the term **head and neck pathology** are used instead, which may indicate that the pathologist deals with otorhinolaryngologic disorders (i.e. ear, nose and throat) in addition to maxillofacial disorders. Oral Pathology is a closely allied speciality with oral and maxillofacial surgery and oral medicine. Oral and maxillofacial pathologist also takes responsibilities in forensic odontology.

Oral pathological warning signs

Because oral health concerns can manifest differently for everyone, it's important to have a specialist experienced in oral pathology diagnose and track their development and progression. For example, some of the common, but often missed, signs of an oral pathological concern may include one or more of the following:

1. Changes in colour in certain areas of tissue

2. Lesions, or bumps, that reappear or don't go away

3. Sores that do not heal quickly, or at all

4. Rough patches or oral tissue

5. Inflammation that doesn't subside

The future of your oral and overall health

Oral pathology includes comprehensive, detailed diagnostic exams and the study of up-to-date oral health records to help better determine the state of your oral and overall health. By understanding these changes and your unique oral health concerns, you can take proper steps to address any potentially serious concerns early and with the right expert treatment.

> There are more bacteria in the human mouth than there are people on the Earth.

Public Health Dentistry

What Does a Public Health Dentist Do?

Dental public health experts provide leadership and guidance in areas such as population-based dentistry, disease prevention, the promotion of dental health, and the surveillance of oral health.

What Is In Toothpaste?

Most toothpastes share common ingredients, both active and inactive. Active ingredients are what help fight cavities and reduce your risk of gum disease. The inactive ingredients give the toothpaste its taste and texture. They may not take an active role in protecting your teeth from cavities or disease, but without them, toothpaste just wouldn't be the same.

Ingredients You Must Know-

Fluoride

When it comes to fighting cavities, fluoride plays a starring role.

It's a mineral that helps strengthen the enamel on your teeth, making them less susceptible to cavities and less likely to wear down from acidic foods and drinks.

Abrasives

Although this ingredient plays an active role in toothpaste, abrasives are technically considered an inactive ingredient because they don't reduce your risk for cavities or gum disease. However, your toothpaste wouldn't have much of an effect without them. Abrasives are the ingredients that remove food debris and stains from teeth.

Flavors

Fluoride and abrasives – these ingredients might help you clean and protect your teeth. What they won't do is taste delicious on their own.

Toothpaste flavours typically come from sweetening agents, such as saccharin or sorbitol. Some toothpaste is even fruit-flavoured for children's use.

Humectants

Some of those flavouring agents, like sorbitol, actually play two roles. Sorbitol is an example of a humectant, an ingredient that prevents the loss of water in toothpaste. A humectant traps water in the toothpaste so that when you squeeze the tube, you get a nice, smooth substance. Along with sorbitol, other examples of humectants include glycol and glycerol.

Detergents

It is important to have detergents in toothpaste because they help foaming to occur when you brush your teeth. One of the most common detergents placed in toothpaste is sodium lauryl sulphate.

How To Choose the Best Toothpaste for You?

When you're looking for toothpaste, you'll find they make various claims about cavity protection, gingivitis, plaque, sensitivity, tartar, whitening and breath-freshening. But for the best protection, find a toothpaste with at least 1,000 parts per million fluoride and the American Dental Association stamp of approval.

Does Whitening Toothpaste Really Work?

It does work but it will cause sensitivity in the long term.

Should I Try An Aloe Vera Toothpaste?

It may reduce plaque and gingivitis but in this paste fluoride content is less which is an essential part of the toothpaste.

What About Charcoal Toothpaste or Powder?

In general, you should avoid charcoal-containing products on your teeth. Charcoal is abrasive, can damage the enamel layer of your teeth and lead to increased long-term sensitivity.

Remember, along with flossing, using good toothpaste is an essential part of your daily dental care routine. The pastes, gels or powders enhance the brushing and cleaning power of the brush. Be sure they contain fluoride so that they will effectively remove plaque, the bacteria film that forms on your gums and teeth after you eat.

Should I Rinse with Water After I Brush?

For any toothpaste, including toothpaste for sensitivity, you reap the benefits by not rinsing after brushing because it will allow the ingredients to be fully absorbed into your teeth and gums. Yet, people usually want to rinse. In addition, sensitive toothpaste typically doesn't taste as good as the regular toothpaste.

Which Toothbrush to Use / Toothbrush Selection

Hard Toothbrush

- Usually not recommended as it may result in abrasion of enamel and gingiva

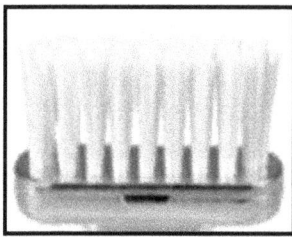

Medium Toothbrush

- Usually recommended for the healthy patient without any gum or dental disease

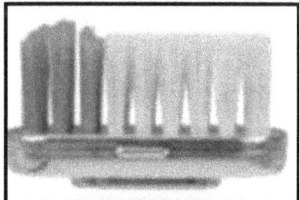

Soft toothbrush (Best for Everyone)

- Patients that apply increased force while brushing
- Patients with gingival recession
- Patients having cervical abrasions

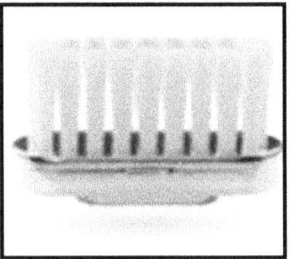

Ultra-Soft Toothbrush

- Patients suffering from severe / desquamative forms of gum disease i.e., painful and bleeding gums with shedding of gums.

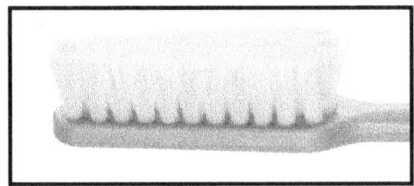

Bamboo toothbrush – has a handle made from bamboo and the bristles are made of nylon. It is a more sustainable and eco-friendly option. It is used in a similar manner as a manual toothbrush.

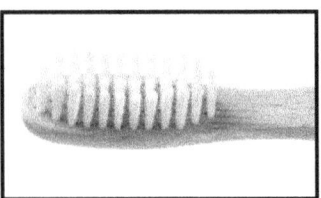

Powered toothbrush – is an electric toothbrush with a wide handle and electrically powered movements of bristles. The larger handle makes it easy to manoeuvre by patients with disability.

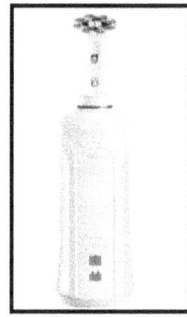

Indications – Patients with mental or physical deficits, hospitalized patients, patients with poor hygiene compliance.

Toothbrushing

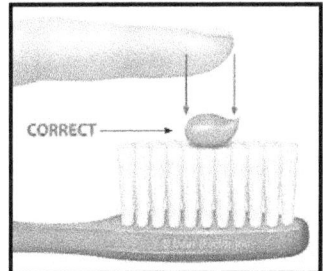
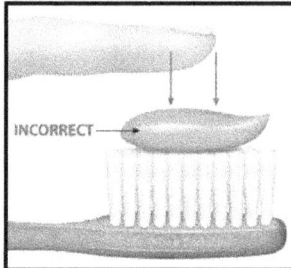

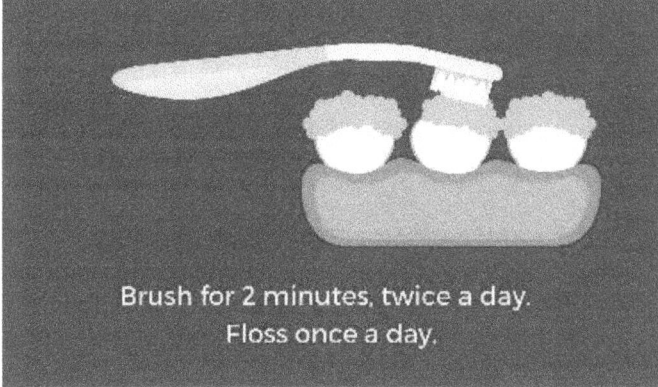
Brush for 2 minutes, twice a day. Floss once a day.

- Use a pea-sized amount of toothpaste
- The duration for brushing teeth should be **2 minutes.** The entire dentition should be divided into 4 parts – upper right, upper left, lower right, and lower left, and each part should be cleaned for **30 secs**. All surfaces including lingual/palatal should be cleaned for all the teeth.
- Should be cleaned under a strong stream of water and another brush may be used to remove the residual bristles.
- It should be stored in open air, allowing proper drying and it should not be in contact with other toothbrushes.
- Toothbrush should be replaced before filaments are frayed, at least every **3 – 4 months.**

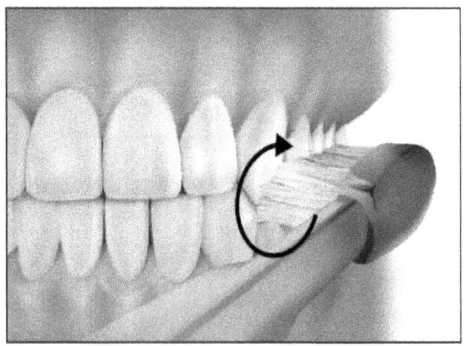

> **Don't smoke or chew tobacco as it is harmful.**

Technique-

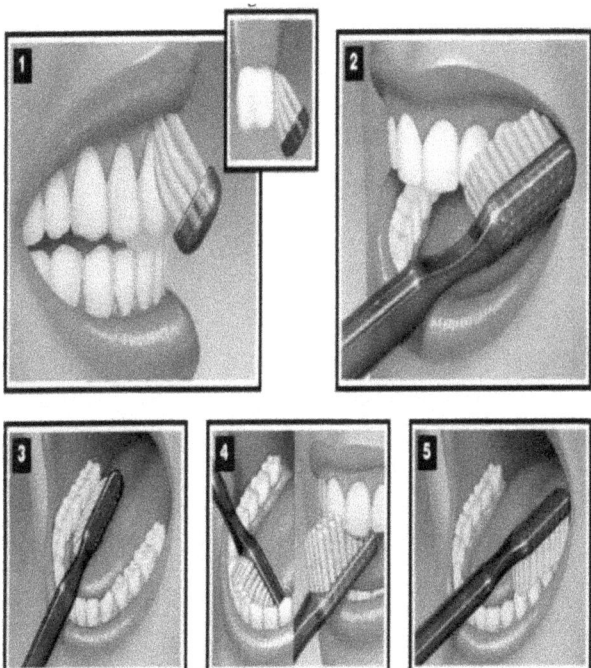

> Don't let the radiance of your smile fade away. Our dental implant specialists can help it shine back.

Lasers in Dentistry

A safer and more comfortable dental treatment for patients.

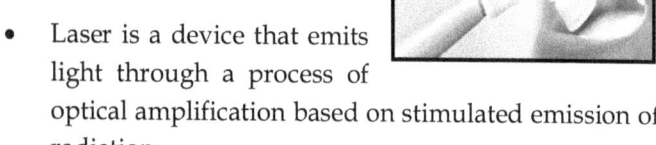

- Laser is a device that emits light through a process of optical amplification based on stimulated emission of radiation

Use-

- For caries removal
- For teeth whitening
- Gum surgery
- RCT
- Frenectomy
- Tongue-its correction

Advantages-

- Less pain.
- Minimizes bleeding.
- Minimizes swelling.
- Reduces anxiety.
- Less damage to surrounding tissues.
- Many procedures do not require anesthesia
- Speeds up healing.

Handy Tips

Bad Breath/ Halitosis

Causes

1. Poor dental hygiene
2. The Coating on the tongue due to poor hygiene
3. Food deposition due to caries or periodontitis
4. Periodontal and oropharyngeal infection
5. Respiratory tract infection
6. Systemic diseases like diabetes, liver and kidney disease
7. External agents like garlic, onion, and smoking

Treatment/ Remedies

1. Diagnosing the cause of halitosis and its treatment. As bad breath may be a result of oral, extraoral, or systemic disease it is necessary to treat the cause.
2. Professional removal of plaque and calculus, followed by proper oral hygiene regime by the patient
3. Use of toothpaste and mouthwashes with odor-masking agents

Sore Throat

Causes

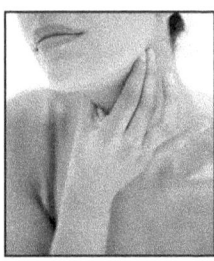

- Viral infection
- Bacterial infection
- Mouth breathing habit
- After the antibiotic course
- After chemotherapy
- Immuno-compromising medications
- Any serious systemic illness

Home Remedies

- Gargling with warm salt water
- Intake of ajwain [herbal remedy] can be helpful
- Tea boiled with basil leaves can also be taken
- Throat lozenges

Sensitive Teeth

Sensitive Teeth

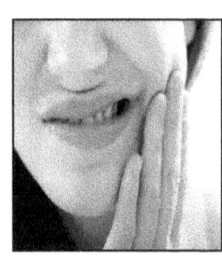

- Brushing hard with pressure in loss of tooth enamel
- excessive sugary content in diet

Home Remedies

- Soft bristle toothbrush
- Avoid drinking too hot or too cold beverages avoid citrus fruit that is acidic
- Avoid the habit of grinding of teeth
- Do not chew tobacco

Dry Mouth

Causes-

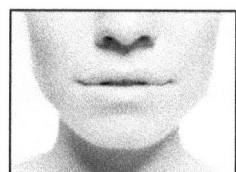

- Auto immune disorders like rheumatoid arthritis, lupus
- chronic aliments like diabetes
- Anemia, anxiety, stress and depression can decrease saliva
- Radiation therapy and other cancer treatment

Home Remedies

- Try sugarless delight [sugarless gum or hard candy that can stimulate salivary gland]
- drink water frequently and avoid aerated drinks
- limit caffeine intake

Avulsed Tooth

Causes

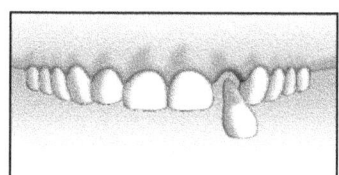

- Falls.
- Bicycle accidents.
- Sports injuries.

- Traffic accidents.
- Assaults.
- Sport injuries

You can put your tooth in:

- A glass of milk.
- A salt solution specifically for preserving avulsed teeth, often found in first aid kids.
- Your cheek, where saliva keeps it wet.
- In saline solution.

Home Remedies

- Pick up your tooth by the crown (white chewing surface). Don't touch the root (the part that usually holds your tooth to the bone below your gumline).
- Rinse your tooth with water or milk to remove any dirt. Avoid using soap, and do not scrub or dry the tooth.
- Gently place your tooth back into the socket, root first. Hold your tooth by the crown and avoid touching the root.
- Bite on a napkin, gauze or handkerchief to anchor your tooth in place.
- Visit a dentist immediately.

Salt Water Rinse

What Does It Do?

The primary benefit of salt water rinse is to reduce bacteria present in the oral cavity and promotes healing.

The primary benefit of salt water rinse is to reduce bacteria present in the oral cavity and promotes healing.

When To Rinse?

2-4 times per day. -The simple salt water mouthwash can help following an extraction, surgery to the gums or tongue, or when a common sore throat or tonsilitis has occurred.

How Does It Work?

"Osmosis attack"

Salt water rinse works against many bacteria by essentially sucking water out of the bacteria which later on kills it.

Simple Recipe-

Use table salt and water

Mix 1 teaspoon of salt (5grams) in 1 cup warm water (250ml)

Pregnancy and Dental

Check-Ups

Pregnancy has 3 trimesters

1 trimester = 0-3 months

2 trimesters = 3-6 months

3 trimesters = 6-9 months

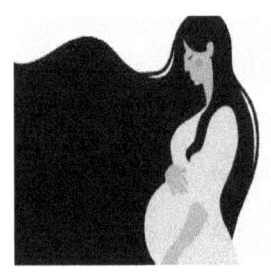

- ✓ **Before**

Keep regular appointments and keep your teeth as healthy as possible.

- ✓ **During**

Make sure your dentist knows you're pregnant.

Inform your dentist of any medications and prenatal vitamins you are taking.

Stick to a balanced healthy diet.

Don't skip your regular dental check-ups.

Rinse your mouth out if morning sickness makes you vomit.

- ✓ **After**

See your dentist to keep your teeth healthy as your body readjusts.

Mouthguards: Things You Need To Know

Due to a sleeping or grinding issue, or because you play a sport, your dentist may recommend a mouthguard to keep your teeth's enamel strong.

Do You Need a Mouthguard?

Mouthguards are an excellent preventive tool for many types of situations that cause harm or injury to your teeth and gums. Even though our enamel, the outermost layer of our teeth, is stronger than bone, damage can occur in several ways. Your dental professional may recommend a mouthguard if you have specific sleep issues or grind your teeth, play sports, or suffer from TMD problems.

How Your Dentist Makes a Mouthguard

A custom-made mouthguard usually involves two appointments with your dental professional. They'll take impressions of your teeth and make a model, sending it to a laboratory where the mouthguard is fabricated for a custom fit. After your mouthguard comes back from the lab, your second appointment is to confirm it fits. Finally, your dental professional will file down any rough edges and make any necessary adjustments for that perfect shape and size, unique to you!

Caring for Your Mouthguard

Just like you clean your teeth every day to remove bacteria, it should be no surprise that you'll need to clean and sanitise your mouthguard after wearing it. It would help if you brushed your guard with a toothbrush and toothpaste after wearing it. Rinse it well, and take time once every week or two to soak it in an antimicrobial solution, such as diluted mouthwash or denture cleaner. Make sure it's dry and store it in a ventilated case. Look for any cracks or rough edges so you won't have a mouthguard that irritates your gums or stores bacteria.

Interesting Teeth and Dental Facts That Will Surprise You

Oral Hygiene and Health

In a lifetime, the average American spends approximately 38.5 total days just brushing their teeth.

It's important to clean your teeth at least twice a day. Not doing so can lead to cavities and gum disease.

Poor dental health can lead to serious health problems such as heart disease and diabetes.

Tooth decay, also known as cavities, is caused by a buildup of plaque on the teeth.

The average woman is more likely than the average man to develop periodontal disease.

Gum disease, also known as periodontitis, is a serious gum infection that damages the soft tissue and can destroy the bone that supports your teeth.

Regular dental appointments are important for maintaining good oral health. Dentists can detect issues early before they become serious, provide necessary cleanings, and give advice on proper oral hygiene practices.

Dental hygienists are essential in maintaining oral health by providing regular cleanings and educating patients on proper oral hygiene.

Americans buy more than 14 million gallons of toothpaste every year.

Coconuts are a natural anti-bacterial food and can help reduce the risk of developing gum disease and cavities.

Approximately 75% of school children worldwide have active dental cavities.

Roughly 25% of American adults have no teeth.

Almost 65 million American adults have some form of periodontal disease. Of this number 38.4% are women, 56.4% are men.

Expectant mothers with poor oral hygiene are 7X more likely to deliver premature and low birth weight babies.

95% of American adults with diabetes also have periodontal disease.

People with periodontal disease are 2X more likely to develop heart disease.

By drinking one can of soda daily, the average American gains 15 lbs each year.

90% of system diseases have oral manifestations.

Kids miss 51 million school hours a year due to dental-related illnesses.

Tooth Anatomy and Material

Here are some interesting facts about teeth

Tooth enamel is the hardest substance in the human body.

The valuable tooth of an elephant, an elephant's molar, is actually made up of a different material, dentin, which is less hard than enamel.

Tooth prints are like fingerprints as they are unique to each person.

Hippopotamuses commonly have 36 teeth. Their dental pattern is composed of two incisors, one canine, three premolars, and three molars, distributed in each quadrant.

Teeth start to form before we are born.

A snail's mouth is no larger than the head of a pin, yet it can contain over 25,000 teeth.

Dental History

During the colonial era, when people lost all their teeth, they frequently resorted to using dentures crafted from ivory or wood.

George Washington's dentures were not made of wood. Rather, he possessed four sets of dentures comprising materials such as gold, ivory, lead, and a blend of human, donkey, and hippo teeth.

The most valuable tooth belonged to Sir Isaac Newton. In 1816 one of his teeth was sold in London for $3,633, or in today's terms $35,700. The tooth was set in a ring!

The first toothbrush was invented by a dentist in China using tufts of wild boar bristles.

The earliest known dentist was Hesi-Ren, an Egyptian who lived thousands of years ago.

False teeth were invented in 1774 by a dentist named Alexis Duchâteau, made from porcelain and animal bone.

There was a unique Victorian tradition of protecting teeth by sealing them with a mixture of ground animal hooves and even turpentine resin.

In ancient times, people believed that baby teeth had protective qualities and they were often used as amulets to ward off evil.

Flossing

Flossing is an essential part of oral hygiene. When you do not floss, you are missing over 40% of tooth surfaces, which is why your dentist always emphasizes flossing!

Although flossing is essential, many people do not like doing it. A whopping 73% of Americans would go to the grocery store than floss their teeth.

The first introduction of commercial floss was in 1882 by Codman and Shurtleff, Inc., later acquired by Johnson and Johnson in 1965.

Floss is also quite durable. A West Virginia inmate once used dental floss to braid a rope, which he used to scale a building and escape in 1992.

In North America, over 3 million miles of dental floss are purchased annually.

Mouth And Saliva Facts

In a lifetime, a person produces over 100,000 gallons of saliva.

One of the most common effects of poor dental hygiene is bad breath. Over 90% of bad breath originates in the mouth.

There are over 700 different types of bacteria in your mouth alone.

Right-handed people tend to chew food on the right side of their mouth, while left-handed people tend to chew their food on the left side of their mouth.

Like your tooth prints and fingerprints, your tongue is also unique. No two people share the same tongue print.

Chewing sugar-free gum can actually be good for your oral health. It helps to clean your mouth and fight off cavities.

Dental Behaviour

25% of adults DO NOT brush twice a day. This increases their risk of developing tooth decay by 33%.

Halloween is the biggest candy-selling holiday, followed by Christmas, Easter, and Valentine's Day.

People who smoke are 2-7 times more likely to develop periodontal disease than non-smokers.

People who drink 3 or more cans of pop daily have 62% more tooth decay, fillings, and tooth loss than people that don't drink pop.

Replacing a toothbrush after illnesses helps prevent the potential for re-infection.

Sweets And Candy

A single can of soda contains 10-12 teaspoons of sugar. The recommended daily dietary intake of sugar is 4 teaspoons.

Sugar Facts: Chemical manufacturers use sugar to grow penicillin. A teaspoon of sugar after a hot curry with extinguish the furnace in your mouth. A spoonful of sugar added to a vase will prolong the life of freshly cut flowers.

Fun And Miscellaneous Facts

Your smile is a strong point of attraction. 61% of adults admit that they are attracted to somebody's smile alone.

The color of your toothpaste apparently matters. More people prefer blue toothpaste over red toothpaste.

A woman smiles, on average, 68 times per day. Meanwhile, a man smiles, on average, eight times per day.

People prefer blue toothbrushes to red ones. The exact reason is unknown, but it could be because blue is often associated with cleanliness.

Did you know that sports-related injuries are a leading cause of chipped teeth? That's why it's always recommended to wear a mouthguard during sporting events.

Fairy floss, also known as cotton candy, was co-invented by a dentist. Despite being mostly sugar, it's not as damaging to teeth as you might think, as it dissolves quickly and doesn't stick to teeth like other sweets.

The common cold can lead to dental problems. Infection in the sinuses, for instance, can cause toothache.

In ancient Assyria, conquered soldiers were expected to clean the king's cats' teeth as part of their duties.

48% of young adults have untagged themselves from a photo on Facebook because of their smile.

It was customary during the middle ages to kiss a donkey if you had a toothache.

It takes 43 muscles to frown. It only takes 17 to smile.

An apple a day may keep the doctor away, but it also makes you 3X more likely to develop dental decay.

According to a recent survey by Time magazine, 59% of people would rather have a dental appointment than sit next to someone who is talking on a cell phone.

Toothpicks are the object most often choked on by Americans.

Sports-related injuries account for approximately 5 million missing teeth per year.

Americans spend $100 billion a year on hair care products, and only $2 billion a year on dental care products.

Every year, kids in North America spend close to half a billion dollars on chewing gum.

The average toothbrush contains about 2500 bristles grouped into about 40 tufts per toothbrush. The tufts are folded over a metal staple and forced into pre-cored holes in the head and fused into the head with heat. The handle is made of at least two materials, usually plastic and rubber. The grips used for the handle are: precision, power, spoon, oblique, and distal oblique.

60% of people don't know that a sore jaw, when combined with chest pain, can signal a heart attack – especially in women.

Americans spent $25 billion on candy in 2010. That is more than the gross national products of Lithuania, Costa Rica, and Mozambique combined.

Dolphins use their teeth to grab only, not to chew, as dolphins' jaws have no muscles.

It generally takes the same amount of time to treat and correct your teeth, regardless of whether you choose Invisalign or traditional braces.

Mosquitoes have 47 teeth.

In 1905, dental assistant Irene Newman was trained to clean teeth. She became the first dental hygienist.

DON'T CRY BECAUSE IT`S OVER,

SMILE BECAUSE IT HAPPENED.

www.ingramcontent.com/pod-product-compliance
Lightning Source LLC
LaVergne TN
LVHW061615070526
838199LV00078B/7293